Intermittent Fasting for Women Over 50

The Simplified Guide to A Fasting Diet Lifestyle with 50 Delicious Low-carb Keto-friendly Recipes

Readers acknowledge that the author is not engaging in the rendering of legal, financial, medical or professional advice.

By reading this document, the reader agrees that under no circumstances are the author or publisher responsible for any losses, direct or indirect, which are incurred as a result of the use of information contained within this document, including, but not limited to errors, omissions, or inaccuracies.

Trademarks

The trademarks that are used are without any consent, and the publication of the trademark is without permission or backing by the trademark owner. All trademarks and brands within this book are for clarification purposes only, and are owned by the owners themselves, who are not affiliated with this document.

TABLE OF CONTENTS

INTRODUCTION

Among the biggest changes that women over the age of fifty experience is a slower metabolism and obesity or increased weight. This is usually associated with the menopause.

In my practice as a nutritionist, I have found that Intermittent Fasting is a good way to reverse and prevent excessive weight gain. Fasting helps to regulate appetite, and when followed regularly, you do not experience the same cravings as other people do. Slower metabolism coupled with less exercise, muscular degeneration and the potential for increased cravings can make it extremely difficult to control weight gain. If you're over fifty and trying to adjust to your slower metabolism, Intermittent Fasting can be of help.

As well as metabolic changes, over fifties begin to experience lower immunity and energy, hence you are at risk of developing chronic diseases like high blood cholesterol and elevated blood pressure (hypertension). In clinical studies, Intermittent Fasting has been shown to decrease the risk of high body cholesterol and blood pressure. If you've noticed a rise in the number of times you've visited a doctor in recent years, it may be time to give Intermittent Fasting a try!

However, Intermittent Fasting may not be suitable for every woman. If you have any health concerns, consult your doctor before starting an Intermittent Fasting diet, especially if you have a condition such as kidney disease or heart disease.

OVERVIEW OF INTERMITTENT FASTING

What is Intermittent Fasting?

It is an eating pattern where one fasts for a particular period of time and then eats for another set of time.

The three most common approaches are: once a week/month, 24 hours and the daily 16/8 or 20/4 intermittent fast. In the 24 hour routine, the individual doesn't eat or drink anything except water, green tea and perhaps some Branched Chain Amino Acids (BCAA) for 24 hours. After the 24 hour period has expired, you begin eating again. During the 16/8 or 20/4 routines, the individual does not eat for either 16 or 20 hours and then eats meals during the remaining 4 to 8 hour period.

Reasons Why You Should Consider Intermittent Fasting Apart From Weight Loss

1. *It reduces your urge to get hungry while dieting.* For someone looking to start dieting, you know that controlling that hunger urge is a massive work to accomplish. But after a few days of starting the Intermittent fasting, your body adjusts to this new eating pattern.

2. *It increases your mental focus and concentration.* As you indulge in fasting, your body releases a chemical called catecholamines (e.g. adrenaline) which significantly increase your mental awareness and your productivity.

3. *It stabilizes your energy levels and improves your mood.* With fewer meals, your blood sugar levels will be kept stable. This will lead to constant energy levels and help you avoid diabetes in the long run.

4. *Reduced oxidative stress.* This simply means that as you fast, it reduces the accumulation of oxidative radicals in the body. This will greatly reduce harm caused to internal organs in your body.

5. *It increases your capacity to resist stress, disease, and aging.* Intermittent fasting, just like exercising, induces a cellular stress response in your body which increases your capacity to cope with stress and resist disease and aging. Recent evidence suggests that it also activates something called "autophagy", which helps your body clear up unwanted and aged parts of cells.

6. *You get to burn fat.* Obviously, this is among the top reasons. You get to lose excess weight. When you eat, your body uses up the glycogen from the food you just ate to give you energy. But as you fast, your body switches to the stored fats and uses them for energy.

7. *It saves you time and money.* Eating fewer meals means preparing and buying fewer meals. Hence you save money and time. Also, you are less exposed to flavors and are therefore less likely to get bored.

How Can You Apply Intermittent Fasting to Your Life?

The best way to apply intermittent fasting to your life is to **start slowly**, and gradually increase the time you do it. This way, you will allow your body to get used to the whole process and you will see results without overwhelming yourself. So, the key is to start slow and gradually increase the amount of time you do it.

The easiest way that my clients find to start is with the 16:8 method, i.e. 16 hours of fasting and 8 hours of feeding. This can easily be adapted to your schedule. See the example schedule below and adapt it for your life.

9am-5pm schedule

Time	Meal
9 am	Breakfast
12 pm	Lunch
4:30 pm	Dinner

Time	Meal
12 pm	Lunch
4 pm	Dinner
7:30 pm	Dessert

In my experience with women over fifty, clients prefer the 12pm-8pm schedule, as they do not tend to miss eating breakfast. However, depending on what your preference is, please adopt what works best for you.

We've designed the recipes in this book to neatly fit into these slots – **Breakfast, Lunch, Dinner and Desserts**. Please prepare and eat one choice from each category. As well as being calorie-controlled, each meal is **keto (low-carb) friendly**, and so this will additionally help you to lose weight. **It's a win-win situation!**

I wish you the best of luck with the recipes in this book, and on your quest for a healthier lifestyle.

BREAKFAST RECIPES

PIZZA RECIPES

Pepperoni Pizza

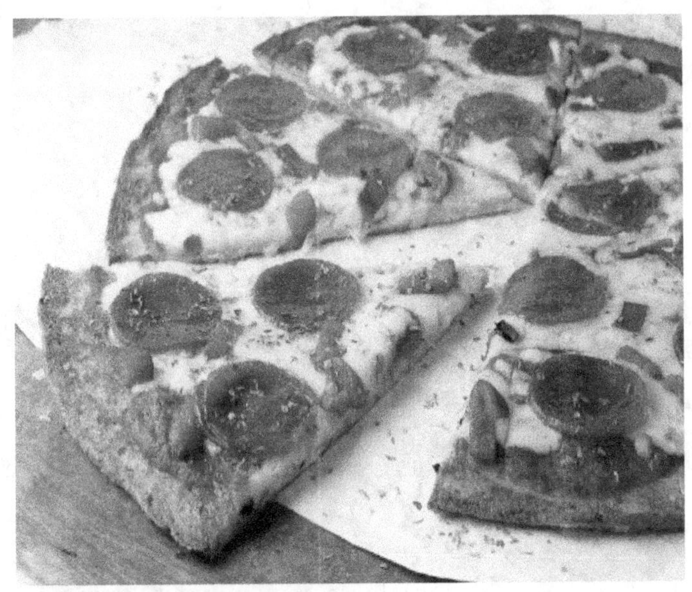

Total Time: 30 minutes

Serves: 2

Ingredients

For the toppings

- 6 slices of pepperoni

- 4 black olives, sliced

- 2 Tablespoons (30 ml) cashew butter

For the base:

- 1/2 cup almond flour

- 2 Tablespoons flax meal

- 1/2 Tablespoon Italian seasoning

- 1 Tablespoons olive oil

- 1 egg

- Salt and pepper, to taste

Instructions

1. Preheat oven to 400 F (200 C).

2. Mix all the base ingredients together to form a dough. Roll out into a round flat pizza crust.

3. Bake for 15 minutes, carefully flipping the crust after 10 minutes.

4. Let the crust cool for a few minutes, then spread the cashew butter on top and top with the pepperoni and olives. Slice the pepperoni into strips if preferred.

5. Place back in the oven for 5 more minutes to crisp up the pepperoni.

Nutrition

- Calories: 470 kcal

- Fat: 41 g

- Net carbs: 5g

- Protein: 16 g

Margherita Pizza

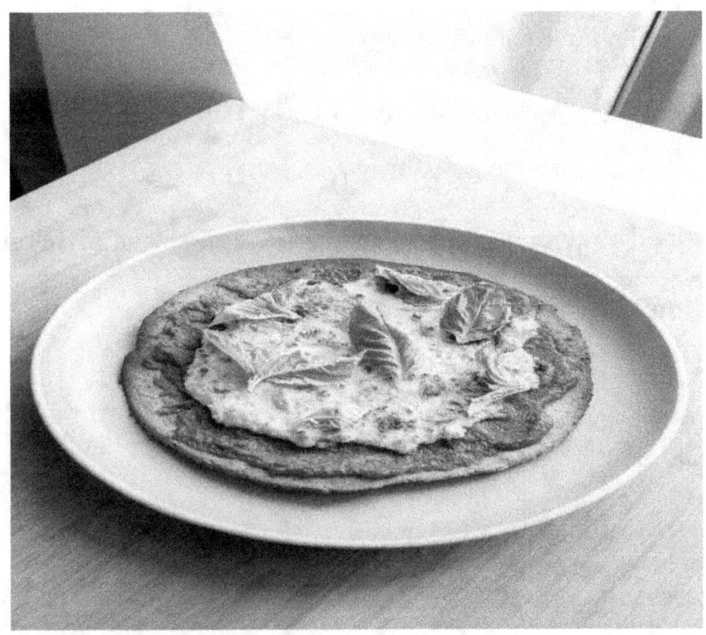

Total Time: 45 minutes

Serves: 4

Ingredients

- 1 Keto almond flour pizza base

- 4 Tablespoons Keto pizza sauce

- 4 Tablespoons Keto cashew cheese (or use cashew or almond butter)

- 6 Basil leaves

- 1 Tablespoon olive oil

Instructions

1. Put together the pizza base.

2. Top with the pizza sauce and cashew cheese.

3. Place back in the oven at 450 F (230 C) for 5-10 minutes until the cheese is browned.

4. Top with basil leaves and a few drizzles of olive oil.

Nutrition

- Calories: 207 kcal

- Fat: 18 g

- Carbohydrates: 7 g

- Protein: 7 g

Vegetarian Pizza

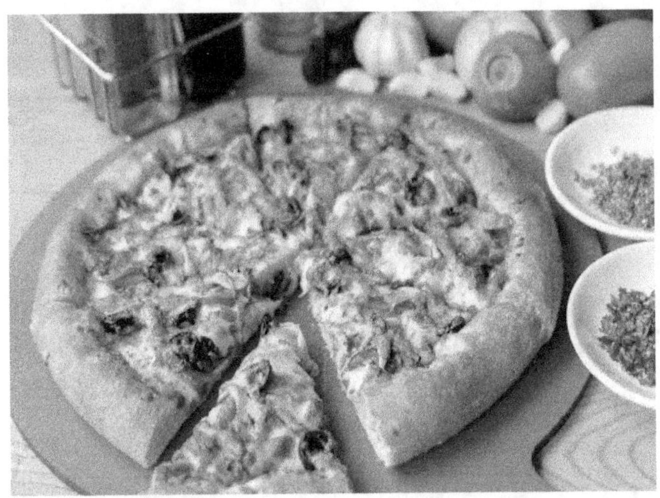

Total Time: 30 minutes

Serves: 4

Ingredients

For the keto pizza crust:

- 1/2 cup almond flour

- 2 Tablespoons flax meal

- 1 Tablespoon nutritional yeast

- 1 Tablespoons olive oil

- 1 egg, whisked

- Salt and pepper, to taste

For the pizza toppings

- 1/4 cup (60 ml) Keto pizza sauce

- 2 Tablespoons (30 ml) cashew butter

- 1 Tablespoon (2 g) nutritional yeast

- 6 basil leaves, chopped

Instructions

1. Preheat oven to 400 F (200 C).

2. Mix all the base ingredients together to form a dough. Roll out into a round flat pizza crust.

3. Bake for 15 minutes, carefully flipping the crust after 10 minutes.

4. Mix the pizza sauce and cashew butter together. Spread on top of the pizza crust.

5. Sprinkle chopped basil on top.

Nutrition

- Calories: 198 kcal

- Fat: 16 g

- Carbohydrates: 8 g

- Protein: 8 g

Cashew Cheese Pizza

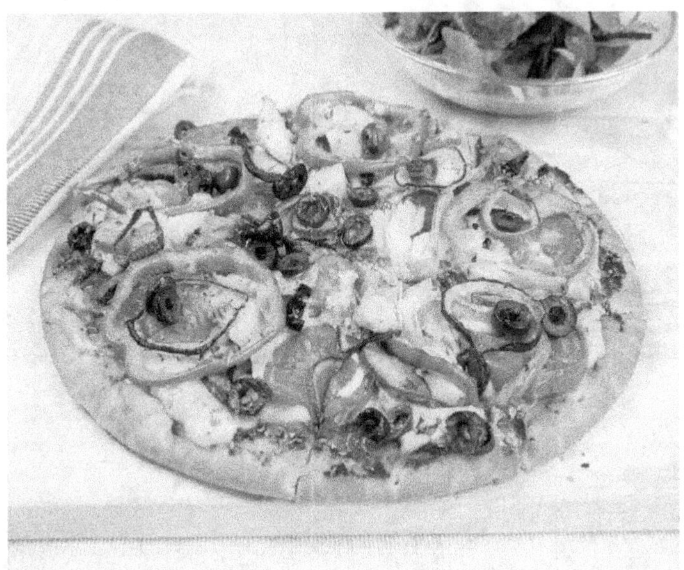

Total Time: 35 minutes

Serves: 4

Ingredients

- 1 Keto pizza crust

- 2 Tablespoons Keto pizza sauce

- 2 Tablespoons cashew cheese

Instructions

- Bake the crust following the instructions.

- Spread 2 tablespoons of Keto pizza sauce on top.

- Then spread the cashew cheese on top.

- Cut into 4 slices and enjoy.

Nutrition

- Calories: 138 kcal

- Fat: 12 g

- Carbohydrates: 5 g

- Protein: 4 g

Cinnamon Pizza

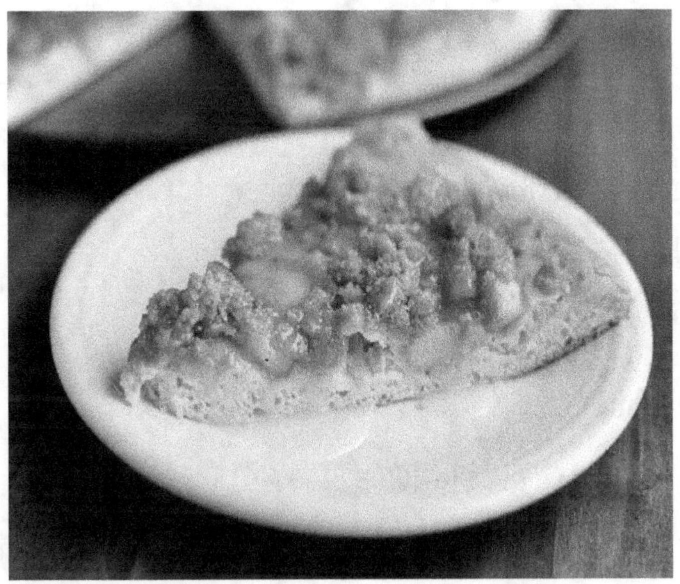

Total Time: 30 minutes

Serves: 8

Ingredients

Pizza base

- 3/4 cup almond flour

- 2 Tablespoons flax meal

- 1 Tablespoon ghee

- 1 teaspoon baking powder

- 1 Tablespoon cinnamon powder

- 1 egg, whisked

* Dash of erythritol, to taste

Cinnamon pizza topping

* 1 Tablespoon ghee, melted

* 1 teaspoon cinnamon powder

Coconut cream topping

* 2 Tablespoons coconut cream

* Erythritol, to taste

Instructions

1. Preheat oven to 400 F (200 C).

2. Mix all the base ingredients together to form a dough. Roll out into a round flat pizza crust.

3. Bake for 15 minutes. Flip and then bake for another 5 minutes.

4. Mix melted ghee and cinnamon together and spread on the pizza crust.

5. Place into freezer for 1 hour to cool down.

6. Mix together the coconut cream and erythritol. Let cool for 30 minutes in the fridge. Spread across the frozen pizza crust.

Nutrition

* Calories: 93 kcal

- Fat: 9 g

- Carbohydrates: 2 g

- Protein: 2 g

LOW-CARB SMOOTHIES

Strawberry Smoothie

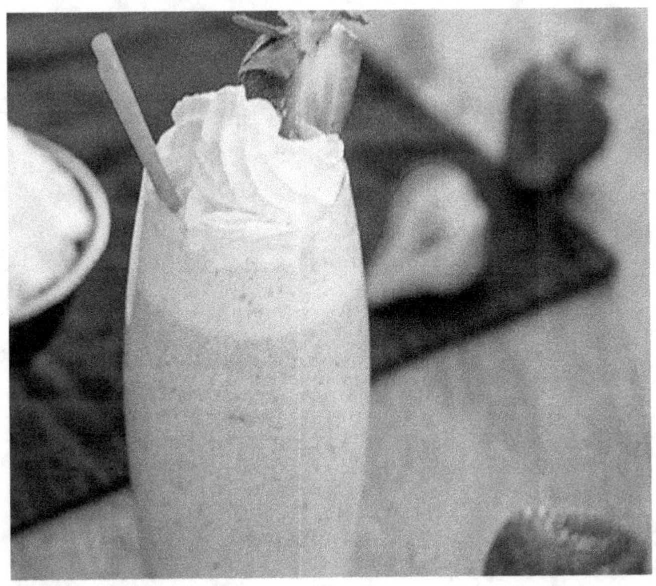

Total Time: 3 minutes

Servings: 1 Smoothie

Ingredients

- 1 1/2 cups unsweetened Almond Milk

- 1 whole Strawberry

- 2 scoops Vanilla Collagen Powder

- 1 tbsp Chia Seeds

- 1 tbsp Heavy Cream

- 2 tsp Vanilla Essence

- 1 tsp Strawberry Essence (optional if you want a stronger

strawberry taste)

- 2 tsp Erythritol (or your choice of sweetener)

Instructions

1. Put all the ingredients into a blender

2. Blend on high until a consistent mixture is achieved

3. For a thicker smoothie allow it to sit for 15 to 30 mins while the chia seeds absorb the liquid

4. Pour into a large glass

5. Enjoy!

Nutrition

- Calories: 332 kcal

- Carbohydrates: 9g

- Protein: 25g

- Fat: 22g

Salted Caramel Smoothie

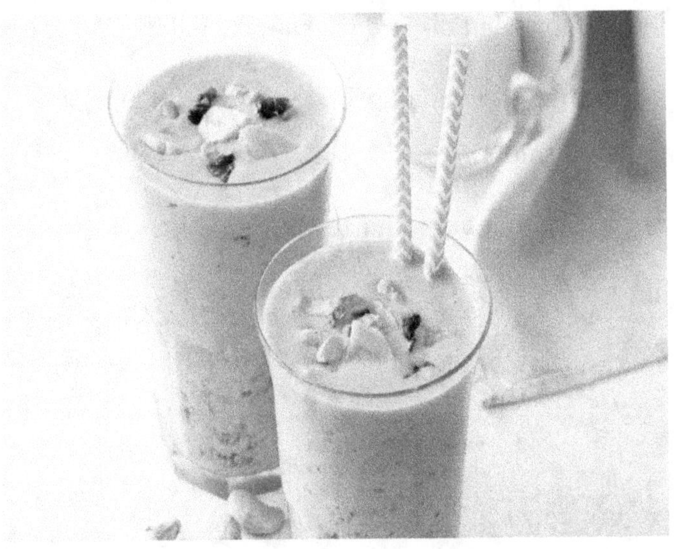

Total Time: 4 minutes

Serves: 1

Ingredients

- 1 bag Bigelow Salted Caramel Tea steeped in 6 oz. water

- 1 cup unsweetened almond milk

- 2 tbsp whipping cream

- 1 tbsp MCT oil

- 1/2 tsp stevia

- 3/4 tsp xanthan gum

- 8 ice cubes

Instructions

1. Steep 1 bag of Bigelow Salted Caramel Tea in 6 oz. water. Remove and discard tea bag when done.

2. Combine remaining ingredients in a blender and blend until smooth.

3. Pour into a glass and serve.

Nutrition

- Calories: 275 kcal

- Fat: 28g

- Protein: 12g

- Carbohydrates: 3g

Acai Almond Butter Smoothie

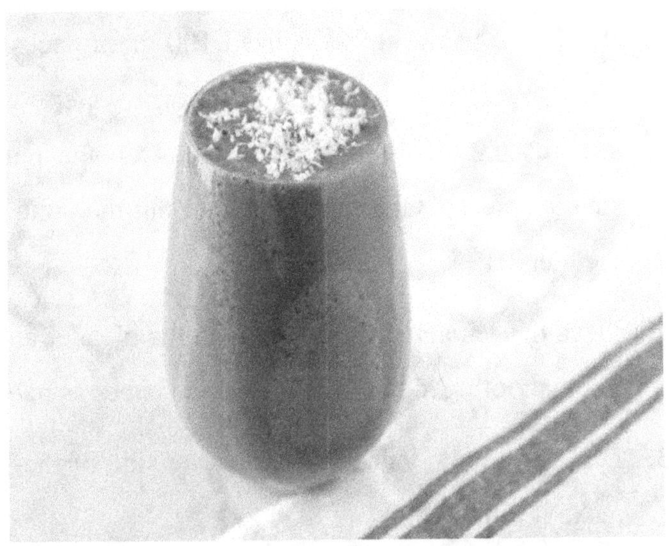

Total Time: 6 minutes

Serves: 1

Ingredients

- 1 100g Pack Unsweetened Acai Puree

- 3/4 cup Unsweetened Almond Milk

- 1/4 of an Avocado

- 3 tbsp Collagen or Protein Powder

- 1 tbsp Coconut Oil or MCT Oil Powder

- 1 tbsp Almond Butter

- 1/2 tsp Vanilla Extract

- 2 drops Liquid Stevia (optional)

Instructions

1. If you are using individualized 100 gram packs of acai puree, run the pack under lukewarm water for a few seconds until you are able to break up the puree into smaller pieces. Open the pack and put the contents into the blender.

2. Place the remaining ingredients in the blender and blend until smooth. Add more water or ice cubes as needed.

3. Drizzle the almond butter along the side of the glass to make it look cool.

4. Enjoy and pat yourself on the back for an awesome workout and killer post workout smoothie!

Nutrition

- Calories: 345 kcal

- Fat: 20g

- Carbohydrates: 8 g

- Protein: 15 g

Blueberry Smoothie

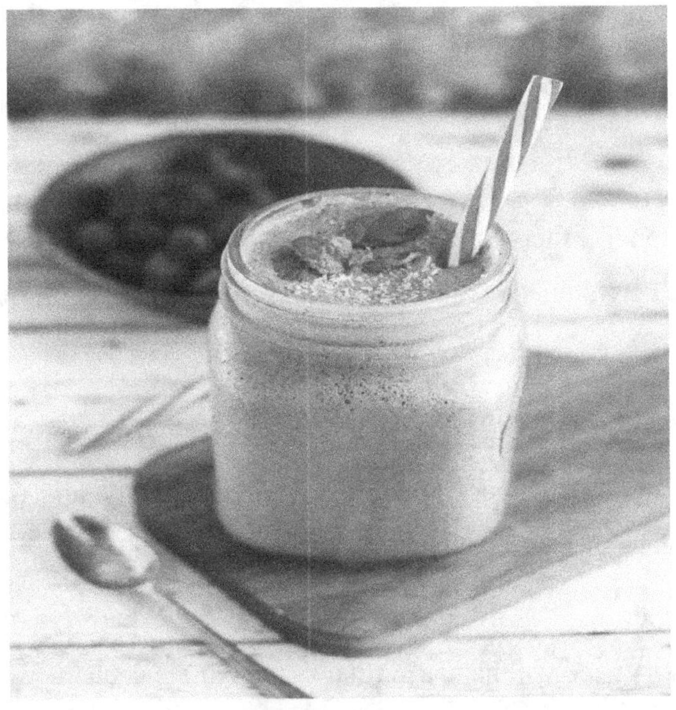

Total Time: 6 minutes

Servings: 1

This keto smoothie is perfect for a quick breakfast or a post-workout refuel option.

Ingredients

- 1 cup Coconut Milk or almond milk

- 1/4 cup Blueberries

- 1 tsp Vanilla Extract

- 1 tsp MCT Oil or coconut oil

- 30 g Protein Powder (optional)

Instructions

1. Put all the ingredients into a blender, and blend until smooth.

Notes

If you like the swirl, you can add a tablespoon of full-fat yogurt after the smoothie was in the cup, and swirled it around, touching the sides.

Suitable Substitutions

MCT Oil - If you don't have any MCT oil that's totally fine, you can replace this with coconut oil, or any fat you like.

Blueberries - Any berry will work (blackberry, raspberry, strawberry) and will have a similar carbohydrate content.

Protein Powder - If you don't have protein powder, you can simply omit this from the recipe. If you still want a fluffy texture, you could try adding a raw egg, but these can sometimes contain salmonella on the eggshell, so pregnant women should avoid this.

Milk Alternatives - you can make it with unsweetened almond milk, unsweetened coconut milk, pea milk, and they all taste similar, just find milk you like, and use that.

Nutrition

- Calories: 215
- Fat: 10g

- Carbs: 7g

- Protein: 23g

Raspberry Avocado Smoothie

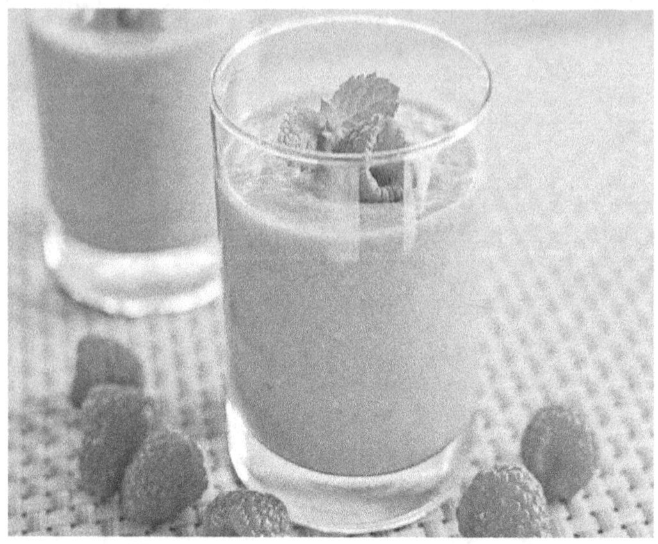

Total Time: 4 minutes

Serves: 2

Ingredients

- 1 ripe avocado peeled and pit removed

- 1 1/3 cup water

- 2-3 tablespoons lemon juice

- 2 Tbsp low carb sugar substitute I like to use 1/8 teaspoon liquid stevia extract

- 1/2 cup frozen unsweetened raspberries or other low carb frozen berries

Instructions

1. Add all ingredients to blender.

2. Blend until smooth.

3. Pour into two tall glasses and enjoy with a straw!

Nutrition

- Calories: 227 kcal

- 4g net carbs

- Fat: 20g

- Protein: 2.5g

OTHER BREAKFAST RECIPES

Almond Pancake

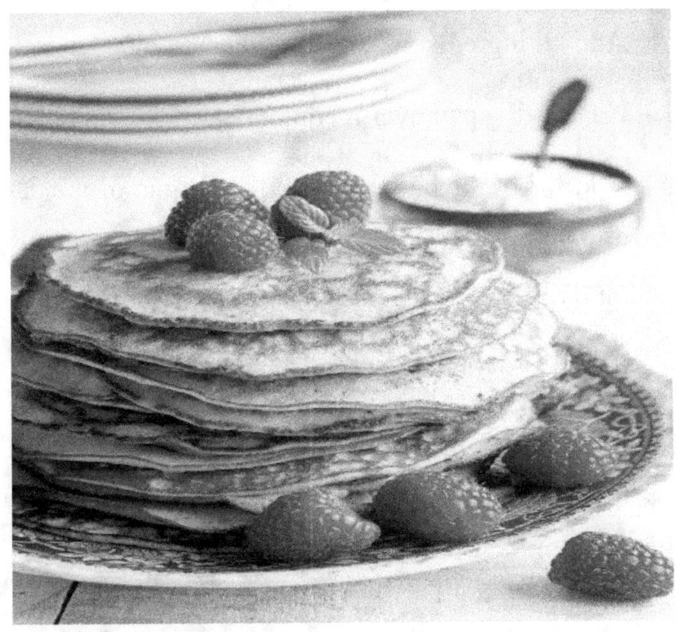

Total Time: 15 mins

Serves: 4

Ingredients

- 1/2 cup Almond Flour
- 1/2 cup Cream Cheese
- 4 Eggs
- 1 tsp Powdered Swerve
- 1 tsp Ground Cinnamon
- 1 tsp Pure Vanilla Extract

- 2 Tbsp Butter (divided - for frying)

Instructions

1. Add all ingredients (except butter) to blender and mix.

2. Heat frying pan over medium heat.

3. Add 1/4 of the butter to coat the bottom of the pan. (Add more butter after frying 2 pancakes. Continue adding butter after every 2 pancakes until batter is gone.)

4. Pour 1/8 of batter (scant 1/4 cup) into the pan.

5. Fry pancakes in melted butter in a non-stick pan over medium heat. Turn over once the middle begins to bubble.

Notes

1. Pancakes should be 4-5 inches in diameter. Serve immediately or store refrigerated in an airtight container for up to one week.

2. After pouring batter into the pan, lift the pan and tilt with a swirling motion to spread the batter until desired pancake size is reached.

3. Be careful not to flip the pancakes too early, they need time to set up while cooking.

4. Serve with sugar-free syrup or, even better, sugar-free lemon curd.

Nutrition

- Calories: 295 kcal

- Fat: 27g

- Carbs: 5g

- Protein: 10g

Chicken Egg Muffins

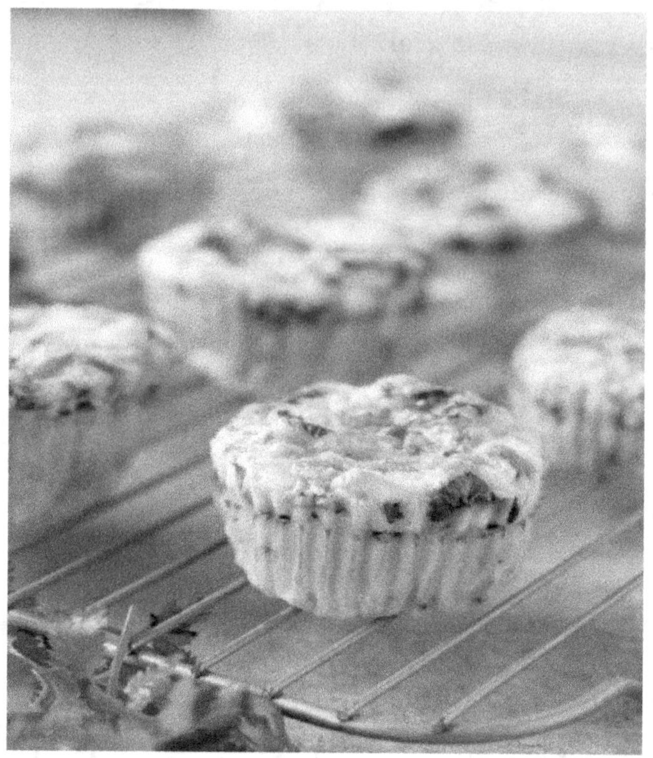

Yield: 12 muffins

Total Time: 30 min

Ingredients

- 11 large eggs

- 1 4-ounce can of green chiles

- 1/2 teaspoon salt

- 1 pinch black pepper

- 1/4 cup mozzarella cheese, shredded

- 1/4 cup cilantro, chopped

- 1/2 cup cooked and shredded chicken

Instructions

1. Preheat oven to 375 degrees. Line a 12-cup muffin pan with parchment paper cup liners and set aside.

2. In a large bowl, whisk together eggs, green chiles, salt, pepper, mozzarella cheese and cilantro. Pour egg mixture evenly into 12 muffin cups.

3. Top each muffin cup with shredded chicken and bake in the oven for 20 minutes.

4. Remove from oven and let rest for at least 5 minutes. Enjoy!

Nutrition

- Calories: 93 kcal

- Fat: 5g

- Carbs 1g

- Protein: 9g

Low-Carb Porridge

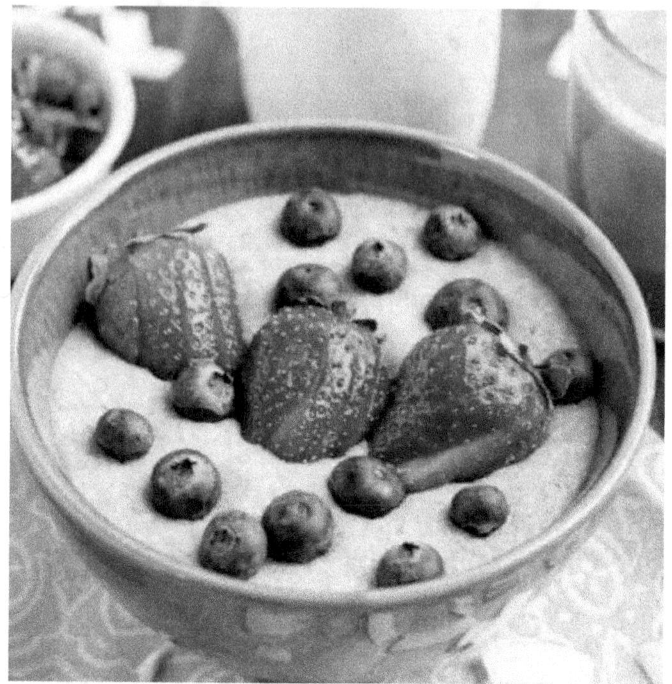

Total Time: 15 minutes

Serves: 6

Ingredients

- 1 cup unsweetened shredded coconut

- 2 cups coconut milk

- 2 2/3 cups water

- 1/4 cup coconut flour

- 1/4 cup whole psyllium husks

- 1 teaspoon vanilla extract

- 1/2 teaspoon cinnamon

- 1/4 teaspoon nutmeg

- 30 drops stevia liquid

- 20 drops monk fruit liquid

Instructions

Instant Pot:

1. Using sauté setting, toast coconut until golden being careful not to burn.

2. Stir in coconut milk and water.

3. Cover. Set on high pressure with timer set to 0 (zero).

4. When time is up, allow a 10 minutes natural pressure release before opening the valve. Open lid and stir in the remaining ingredients.

Stove Top:

1. In medium pot over medium high heat, toast coconut being careful not to burn.

2. Stir in coconut milk and water.

3. Cover and bring to a boil.

4. After reaching a boil, remove from heat and stir in the remaining ingredients.

Nutrition

- Net Carbs: 5g

- Calories: 303 Kcal

- Fat: 25g

- Carbohydrates: 9g

- Protein 3g

Cauliflower Toast With Avocado

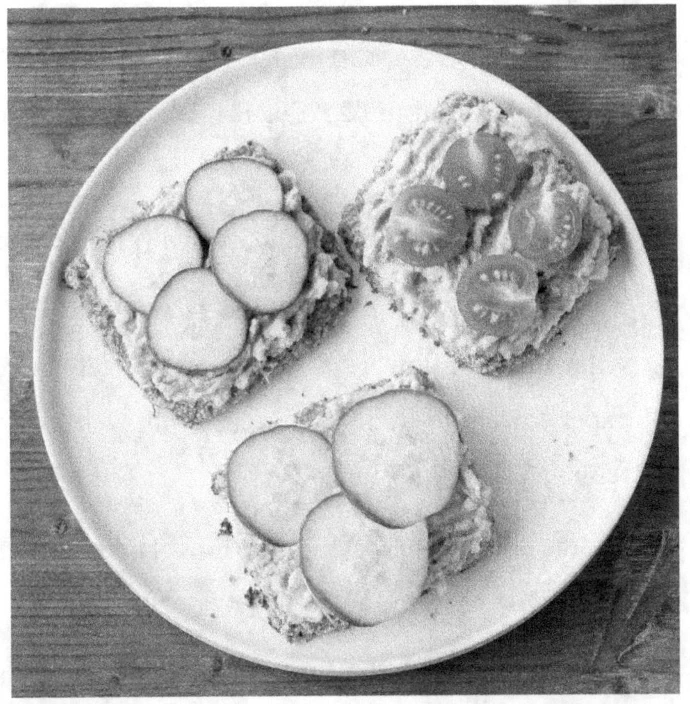

Serves: 2

Total Time: 30 minutes

Ingredients

- 1 small head cauliflower (grated)

- 1 large egg

- 1/2 cup mozzarella cheese

- 1/2 teaspoon garlic powder

- 1 medium avocado (pitted and chopped)

- 1 tablespoon fresh lime juice

- salt and pepper

Instructions

1. Preheat the oven to 425°F and line a baking sheet with parchment or foil.

2. Place the cauliflower in a microwave-safe bowl and heat on high for 8 minutes.

3. After the cauliflower has cooled completely, spread on paper towels to drain and press with a clean towel to remove excess moisture.

4. Put the cauliflower back in the bowl and stir in the egg, mozzarella cheese, and garlic powder.

5. Season with salt and pepper and stir until well combined.

6. Spoon the mixture onto the baking sheet in four rounded squares, as evenly as possible.

7. Bake for 18 to 20 minutes until golden brown on the edges.

8. Mash the avocado with the lime juice and a pinch of salt and pepper.

9. Spread the avocado onto the cauliflower toast to serve. Makes 2 servings.

10. For leftovers, prepare the cauliflower toast as directed and prepare the avocado mash fresh.

Nutrition

- 300 Calories

- 23.5g of Fat

- 10g of Protein

- 6.5g of Net Carbs

Zucchini Pizza Boats

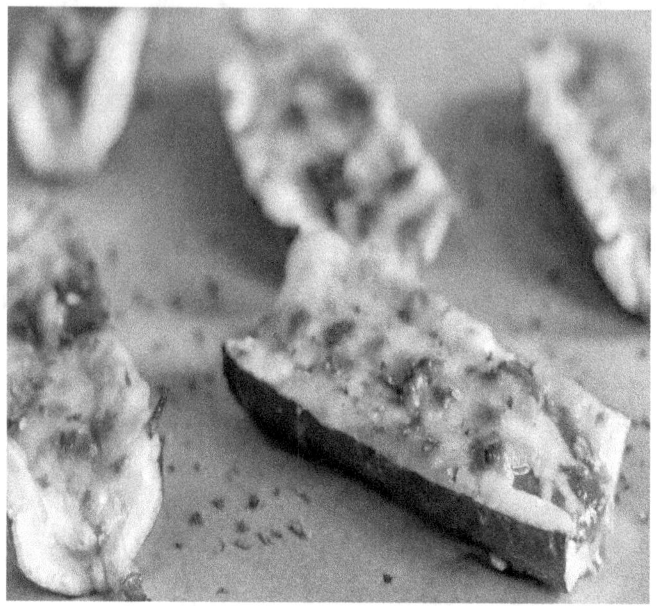

Make easy Zucchini Pizza Boats in the Air Fryer. These are low-carb and keto-friendly!

Total Time: 13 min

Yield: 8

Ingredients

- 2 Zucchini (More if they are small)

- 1/4 Cup Pizza Sauce

- Mini Pepperoni

- Shredded Mozzarella Cheese

- Olive oil spray

Instructions

1. Cut the zucchini in half if they are long and then again lengthwise.

2. Scoop the middle portion out with a spoon.

3. Spray the zucchini lightly with olive oil spray.

4. Add in the pizza sauce, top with pepperoni and cheese.

5. Place them in the air fryer basket.

6. Coat with an even coat of olive oil spray.

7. Air fry at 350 degrees for 8 minutes.

8. Add an additional 2 minutes if needed to crisp the cheese.

9. Repeat if necessary for the additional zucchini.

Nutrition

- Calories: 61 kcal

- Total Fat: 4g

- Carbs: 3g

- Protein: 2.4g

Air Fry Olive Bread

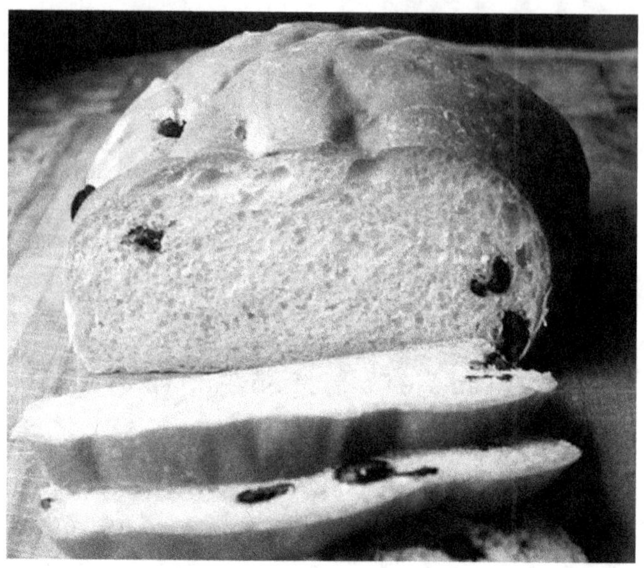

Cook Time: 30 minutes

Servings: 6

Ingredients

- 1 cup + 2 table spoon Almond Flour

- 1 tsp Baking Powder

- 1/4 tsp Salt

- 1/4 tsp Baking Soda

- 1 tsp Monk Fruit Sweetener granules

- 1/4 cup Flaxseed Meal

- 1 large Egg

- tablespoons olive oil

- 1/3 cup Black Olives chopped coarsly

- 1 tablespoon Water

Instructions

1. Prepare an Air Fryer cooking pan with cooking spray so the bread dough does not stick.

2. In a large bowl mix all the ingredients together until well combined.

3. Shape the dough into a round loaf (or shape of choice) and put it inside the pan. Place the pan inside the Air Fryer and cook on the bread/cake setting. (Should be 330 degrees for about 30 minutes on the Air Fryer, some temps may vary)

4. Cook the bread until the timer goes off. The bread should rise a bit and be completely dry on the top and bottom of the loaf. (If not you can cook a bit longer)

Nutrition

- Calories: 256 kcal

- Fat: 23.6g

- Protein: 6.4 g

- Net Carbs: 2.4 g

LUNCH RECIPES

AIR-FRYER RECIPES

Chicken Thighs With Adobo Seasoning

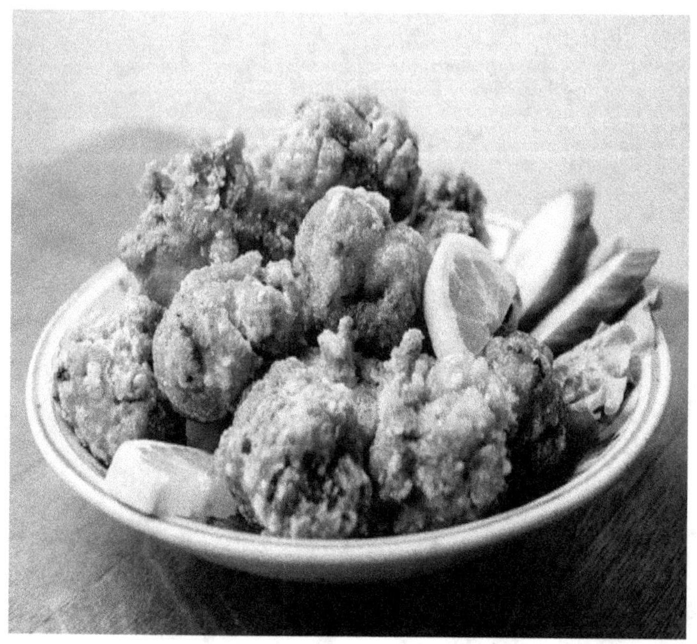

Total time: 25 min

Serves: 4

Ingredients

- 4 large chicken thighs

- 2 tbsp adobo seasoning (Use Light or Low Sodium Adobo seasoning if you like chicken less salty)

- 1 tbsp olive oil

Instructions

1. Add olive oil to bag or plate and coat chicken in it.

2. Toss chicken thighs in adobo seasoning to coat.

3. Place chicken thighs in air fryer basket, making sure they don't touch or crowd each other.

4. Set air fryer to 350 degrees and set the timer to 10 minutes.

5. After 10 minutes, flip chicken to other side and cook another 10 minutes.

6. Chicken will be golden brown and 165 degrees internal temperature at the end of cooking.

Nutrition

- Calories: 340 kcal

- Carbs: 2g

- Fats: 14g

- Protein: 26g

Four-Ingredient Keto Wings

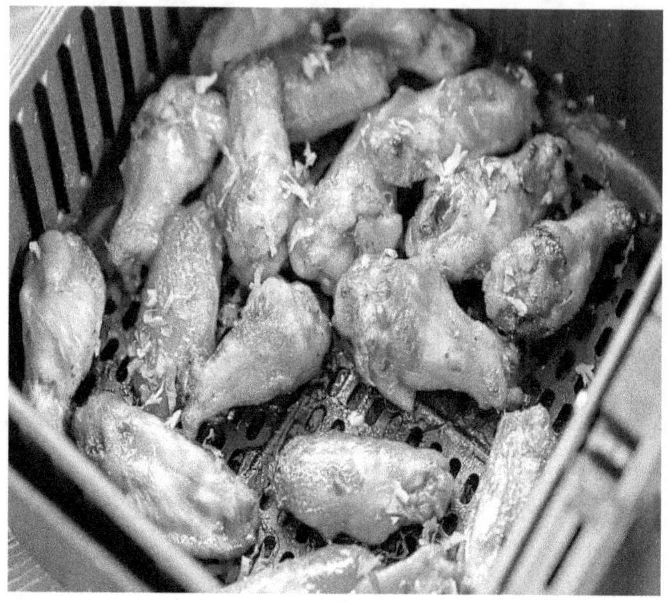

Make crispy, crowd-pleasing wings in the air fryer with very little effort!

Serves: 4

Total Time: 37 min

Ingredients

- 12 chicken wings, uncooked

- salt & pepper to taste

- 1 tablespoon olive oil spray

- 3 tablespoons buffalo chicken wing sauce

Directions

1. Simply place raw chicken wings in air fryer basket. Salt & pepper to taste. Mist with cooking spray.

2. Set the timer for 30 minutes at 370 degrees Fahrenheit.

3. At the halfway mark, turn them and mist the wings with cooking spray.

4. Once they are done cooking to your desired crispness, toss with wing sauce and enjoy!

5. Note: Refer to the next recipe (on page 103) for the buffalo sauce recipe!

Nutrition

- Calories: 273 kcal
- Total Carbohydrates:0g
- Total Fat: 20g
- Protein: 22g

Chicken Hot Wings With Buffalo Sauce

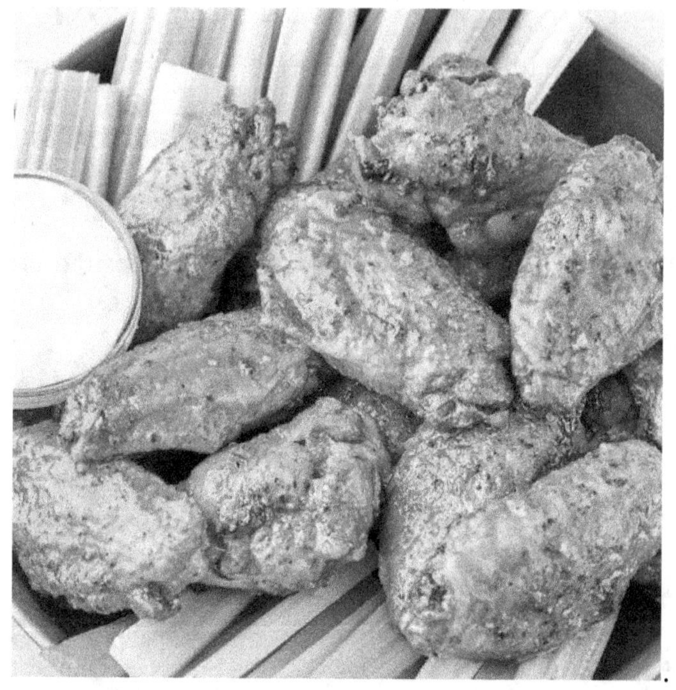

Total Time: 34 minutes

Servings: 5 people

Ingredients

Wings

- 2 pounds chicken wingettes

- 1 tablespoon olive oil or avocado oil

- 1/2 teaspoon garlic powder

- 1/2 teaspoon salt

- extra oil for greasing

Buffalo Sauce

- 1/3 cup hot pepper sauce (You can use Frank's Red Hot)

- 1/4 cup butter butter flavored coconut oil for dairy-free

- 1 tablespoon white vinegar

- 1/8 teaspoon ground chipolte pepper or cayenne pepper

Instructions

For the Buffalo Sauce:

1. While wings are cooking in air fryer, combine hot sauce, butter, vinegar, and ground pepper in small pot.

2. Bring sauce to a boil on medium heat while whisking everything together. Remove from heat and set aside.

3. When wings are done, add them to the sauce and coat each piece evenly.

4. Serve with blue cheese dressing and celery.

Wings:

1. In large bowl, rub olive oil on chicken wings and then sprinkle on the garlic powder and salt.

2. Rub inside of air fryer basket with a little more olive oil, avocado oil, or coconut oil.

3. Place chicken wings in a single layer in basket.

4. Cook wings at 360°F for 25 minutes.

5. Flip wings over. Then increase temperature to 400°F and cook for 4 more minutes.

Nutrition

- Calories: 327kcal

- Carbohydrates: 0g

- Protein: 18g

- Fat: 27g

Buttermilk Fried Chicken

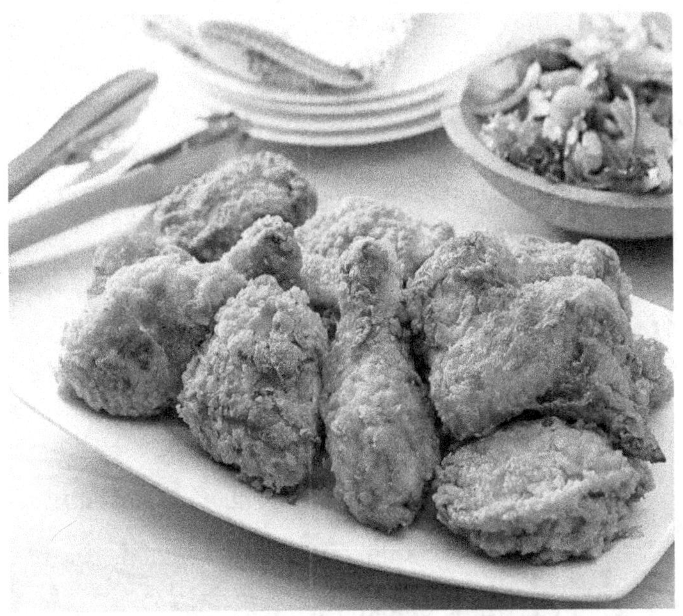

This awesome recipe is a traditional, Southern soul food recipe. This dish is quick to whip up, with less than 7 ingredients. The results are crispy, crunchy fried wings.

Total Time: 30 minutes

Servings: 5

Ingredients

- 2 1/2-3 pounds whole chicken wings

- 1/4 cup buttermilk

- 3/4 cup almond flour

- McCormick's Grill Mates Montreal Chicken seasoning,

to taste

- salt and pepper to taste

- cooking oil

Instructions

1. Add the chicken wings to a large bowl. Drizzle with the buttermilk.

2. Combine almond flour, chicken seasoning, salt and pepper in a bowl large enough to dredge the chicken. Stir and mix well.

3. Dredge the chicken in the flour and seasonings. Ensure both sides of the chicken are fully coated. Use a spoon to get areas of the chicken wing that were missed.

4. Spray the air fryer basket with cooking oil.

5. Add the chicken wings to the air fryer. It's ok to stack the chicken, but do not overcrowd the basket. Cook in batches if necessary

6. Cook for 20 minutes on 400 degrees. Stop and flip the chicken every 5 minutes, a total of 4 times.

7. Ensure the chicken is cooked on the inside. Use a meat thermometer and ensure the chicken has reached an internal temperature of 160 degrees. Add additional time if you prefer the chicken is crisper.

8. Remove from the air fryer. Cool before serving.

Nutrition

- Calories: 240 kcal

- fats: 14g

- sugars: 0.5g

- protein: 18g

Gochujang Chicken Wings (Korean Recipe)

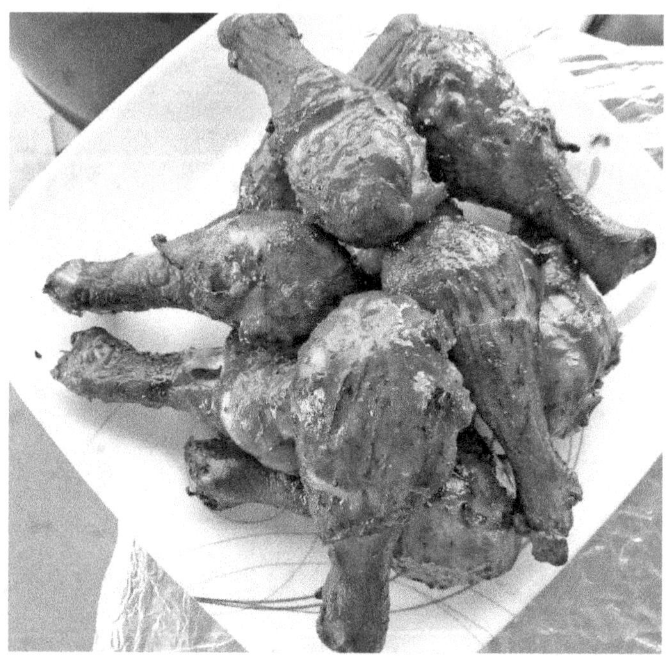

Total Time: 40 minutes

Servings: 4

Ingredients

For the Wings:

- 2 pounds chicken wings

- 1 teaspoon Salt

- 1 teaspoon Ground Black Pepper, or gochujaru

For the Sauce:

- 2 tablespoons gochujang

- 1 tablespoon mayonnaise

- 1 teaspoon agave nectar

- 1 tablespoon Sesame Oil

- 1 tablespoon minced ginger

- 1 tablespoon Minced Garlic

- 1/3 cup stevia

For Finishing:

- 2 teaspoons Sesame Seeds, optional

- 1/4 cup Green Onions, optional

Instructions

1. Preheat your air fryer to 400°F

2. Salt and Pepper the chicken wings and place in the air fryer basket.

3. Set the timer to 20 minutes and allow the chicken wings to cook, turning once at 10 minutes.

4. As the chicken bakes or air fries, mix together all the sauce ingredients and let the sauce marinate while the chicken wings finish cooking.

5. As you near the 20-minute mark use a thermometer to check the meat. When the chicken wings reach 160F

remove them from the oven and place into a bowl.

6. Pour about half the sauce on the wings, and toss to coat the wings with the sauce.

7. Place the chicken wings back into the oven or air fryer and cook for another 5 minutes until the sauce has glazed over, and the chicken is completely cooked and has reached at least 165F.

8. Remove, sprinkle with sesame seeds and chopped green onions and serve!

Nutrition

- Calories: 356 kcal

- Carbohydrates: 6g

- Protein: 23g

- Fat: 26g

Almond Flour Air Fried Chicken

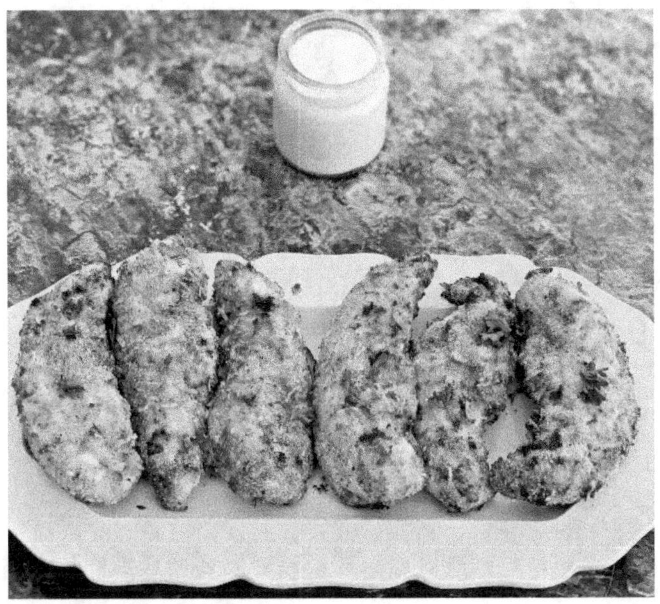

Total Time: 22 minutes

Servings: 4

Ingredients

- 4 Chicken Breasts, about 4 ounces each and pounded to an even thickness. About 1/3 inch is thickness is best.

- 1 cup Almond Flour

- 1/2 cup Parmesan Cheese

- 1 tsp. Garlic Powder

- 1 tsp. Onion Powder

- 1 tsp. Paprika

- 2 tsp. salt

- 1 tsp. pepper

- 1 egg beaten

Instructions

1. Trim and pound the chicken breasts. A thickness of 1/3 of an inch is best.

2. Salt and pepper the outside of the chicken and set aside.

3. Mix the egg up in a dish. Be sure it's one your chicken will fit into as you'll be dipping the chicken in the egg first.

4. In another dish mix together almond flour, parmesan cheese, garlic powder, onion powder, paprika, salt and pepper.

5. Dredge the chicken in the egg and then the almond flour mixture.

6. Preheat your air fryer to 390 degrees. Just allow it to run for 2-3 minutes.

7. Spray the air fryer basket with cooking spray. Add the chicken, then spray the tops of the chicken with cooking spray as well.

8. Air fry for 10-12 minutes or until the chicken reaches an internal temperature of 165 degrees. Flip it halfway through cooking. I like to use an instant read thermometer

to check my chicken. It's easy to overcook it when air frying.

Nutrition Facts

- Calories: 248 Kcal

- Fat: 11.3g

- Carbs: 5g

- Protein: 33g

Crispy Cod

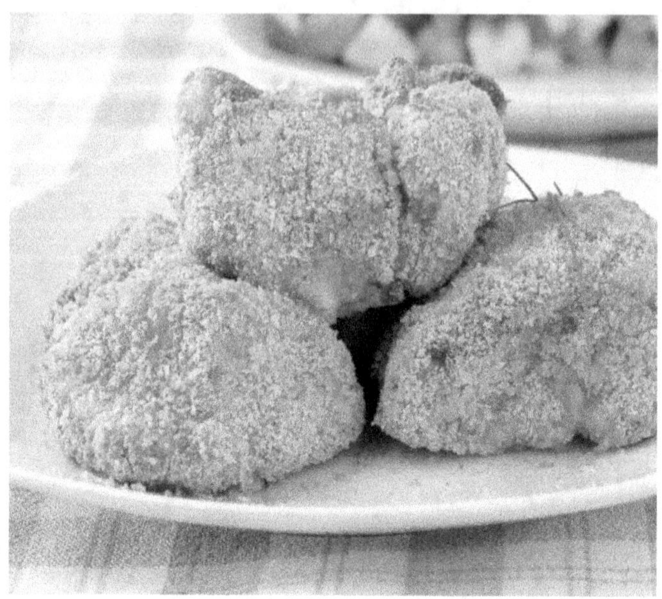

Total Time: 15 mins

Servings: 2

Ingredients

- 1 lb cod fillet
- 1 lemons
- 1/4 cup butter
- 1 tsp salt
- 1 tsp seasoning salt

Instructions

1. Prepare ingredients for the air fryer cod fillets. Season

fillets with your favorite seasoning.

2. Brush the air fryer basket with oil. Place fillets in the basket. Top it off with butter and lemon slices.

3. Cook cod in the air fryer at 400°F for 10-13 minutes, depending on the size of fillets. The internal temperature should reach 145°F.

Nutrition

- Calories: 405 kcal

- Fat: 25g

- Carbs: 5g

- Protein: 41g

Cajun Shrimp

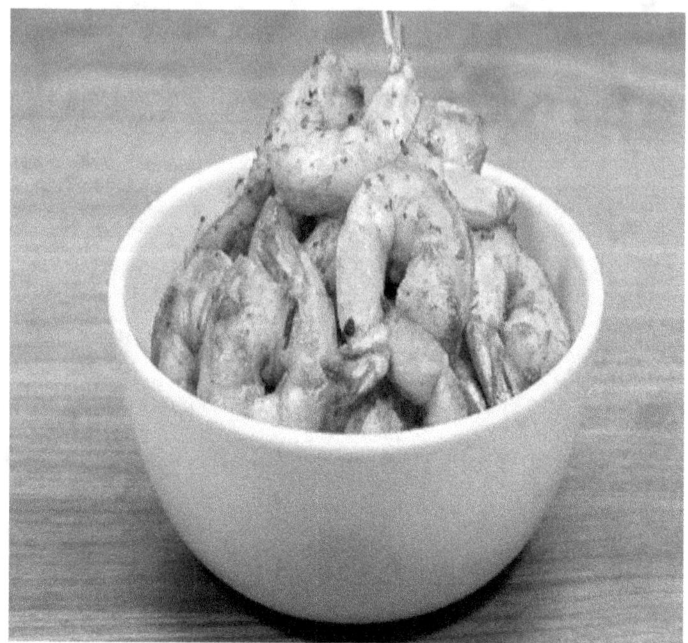

Total Time: 30 mins

Servings: 3

Equipment: Airfryer

Ingredients

- 1 tablespoon Cajun or Creole seasoning

- 24 (1 pound) cleaned and peeled extra jumbo shrimp

- 6 ounces fully cooked Turkey/Chicken Andouille sausage or kielbasa, sliced

- 1 medium zucchini, 8 ounces, sliced into 1/4-inch thick half moons

- 1 medium yellow squash, 8 ounces, sliced into 1/4-inch thick half moons

- 1 large red bell pepper, seeded and cut into thin 1-inch pieces

- 1/4 teaspoon kosher salt

- 2 tablespoons olive oil

Instructions

1. In a large bowl, combine the Cajun seasoning and shrimp, toss to coat.

2. Add the sausage, zucchini, squash, bell peppers, and salt and toss with the oil.

3. Preheat the air fryer 400F.

4. In 2 batches (for smaller baskets), transfer the shrimp and vegetables to the air fryer basket and cook 8 minutes, shaking the basket 2 to 3 times.

5. Set aside, repeat with remaining shrimp and veggies.

6. Once both batches are cooked, return the first batch to the air fryer and cook for 1 minute.

Nutrition

- Calories: 284 kcal

- Carbs: 8g

- Protein: 31g

- Fat: 14g

Italian Pork Chops Recipe

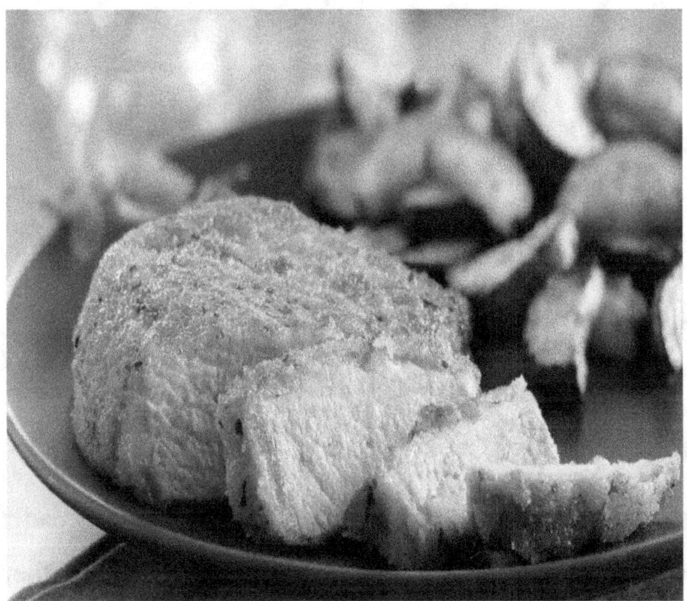

Total Time: 28 mins

Serves: 3

Ingredients

- 3 (6 oz.) pork chops, rinsed & patted dry

- salt, to taste

- black pepper, to taste

- garlic powder, to taste

- smoked paprika, to taste

- 1/2 cup panko breadcrumbs

- 1/2 cup grated parmesan cheese

- 2 Tablespoons chopped Italian parsley, plus more for optional garnish

- 1 large egg

- Cooking spray, for coating the pork chops

- 1/2 cup grated mozzarella cheese

- 1 cup marinara sauce, heated

Directions

1. Season the pork chops with salt, pepper, garlic powder, and smoked paprika.

2. In medium bowl, mix together the panko breadcrumbs, parmesan cheese, and chopped parsley. In another bowl, beat the egg.

3. Dip each pork chop in egg and then dredge it in the breadcrumb mixture, coating completely. Lightly spray both sides of coated pork chops with cooking spray right before cooking.

4. Preheat the Air Fryer at 380°F for 4 minutes.

5. Place in the Air Fryer and cook at 380°F (194°C) for 8-12 minutes. After 6 minutes of cooking, flip the pork chops and then continue cooking for the remainder of time or until golden and internal temperature reaches 145-160°F.

6. Top with cheese and air fry for 2 more minutes to melt

the cheese.

7. Serve warm with marinara sauce.

Nutrition Facts

- Calories: 326 kcal

- Fat: 18g

- Carbs: 4g

- Protein 32g

Spicy Green Beans

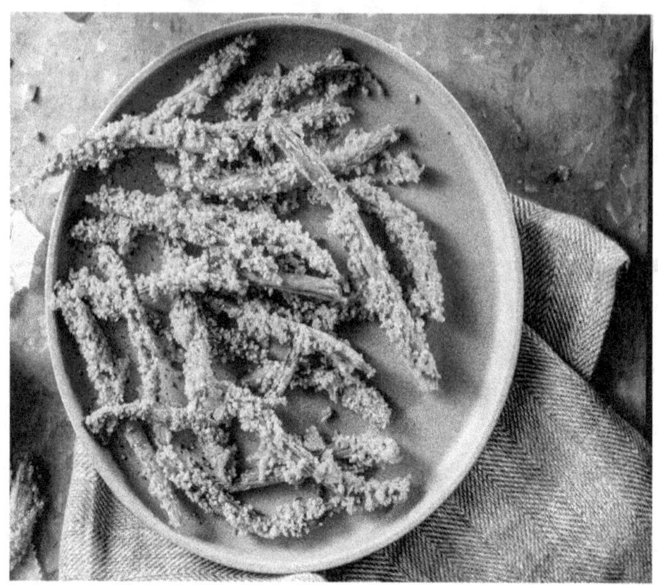

Total Time: 20 min

Serves: 4

Ingredients

- fresh green beans (trimmed)

- 12 oz olive oil

- 1 tbsp Thai-style chili garlic paste

- 1 tsp panko bread crumbs

- 1 tbsp salt

Directions

1. Place the green beans in a medium bowl and toss with the

olive oil, chili garlic paste, panko bread crumbs, and salt.

2. Place the green beans in the air fryer basket. Set the temperature to 400° F and air fry for 4 minutes. Shake the air fryer basket. Air fry for an additional 5 to 7 minutes. Serve warm.

Nutrition Facts

- Calories: 60 kcal

- Total Fat: 3.5g

- Carbs: 1g

- Protein 2g

OTHER LUCH RECIPES

Creamy Chicken Lettuce Cups

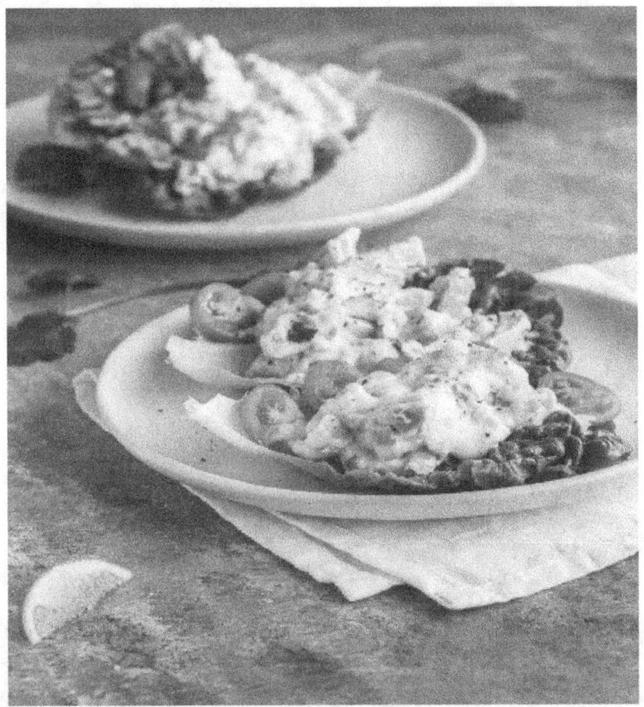

Total Time: 30 minutes

Servings: 1

Ingredients:

- 1 Medium Chicken Breast (4 oz)

- 3 Large Lettuce Leaves

- 3 Cherry Tomatoes

- 1 Tbsp Red Onion

- 3 Tbsp Homemade Mayonnaise

- 1 Tbsp Corriander (cillantro)

- 1 Tbsp Sesame Seed Oil

- dash Salt and Pepper

Instructions

1. Place the chicken breast on a baking tray, cover with some sesame seed oil and bake for 20 mins at 180C (355F)

2. Cut the 3 large leaves of lettuce from the stalks to make cups (Iceberg works best)

3. Slice the tomatoes and red onion, placing them in each lettuce cup.

4. Remove the chicken from the oven and slice into small strips.

5. Mix the mayonnaise with the coriander, add a little sesame seed oil and drop over the lettuce cups. Cover with salt and pepper.

Nutrition

- Calories: 499 kcal

- Fat: 32g

- Carbs: 10g

- Protein: 40g

Broiled Chicken & Artichokes

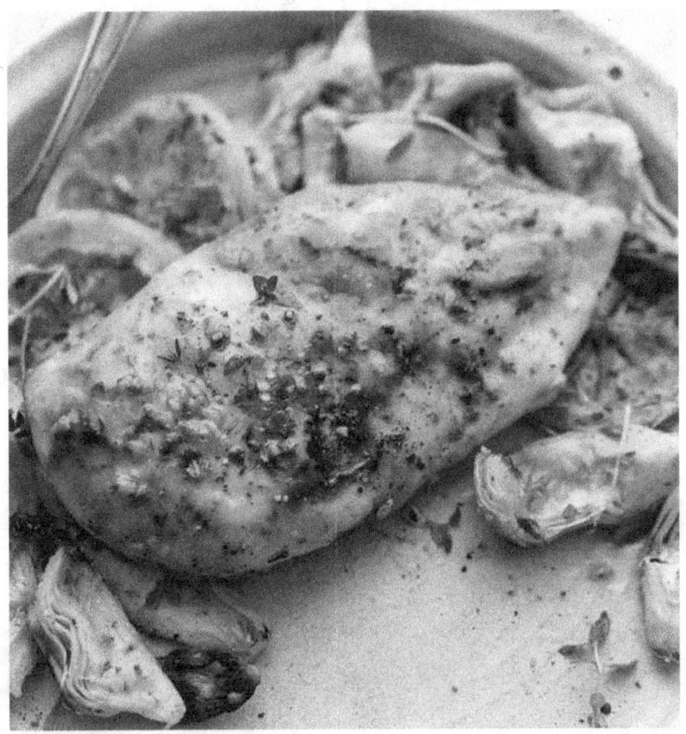

Total Time: 15 min.

Serves: 8

Ingredients

- 8 boneless skinless chicken thighs (about 2 pounds)

- 2 jars (7-1/2 ounces each) marinated quartered artichoke hearts, drained

- 2 tablespoons olive oil

- 1 teaspoon salt

- 1/2 teaspoon pepper

- 1/4 cup shredded Parmesan cheese

- 2 tablespoons minced fresh parsley

Instructions

1. Preheat boiler. In a large bowl, toss chicken and artichokes with oil, salt and pepper. Transfer to a broiler pan.

2. Broil 3 in. from heat 8-10 minutes or until a thermometer inserted in chicken reads 170°, turning chicken and artichokes halfway through cooking. Sprinkle with cheese. Broil 1-2 minutes longer or until cheese is melted. Sprinkle with parsley.

Nutrition

- Calories: 288 kcal

- 21g fat

- 4g carbohydrate

- 22g protein.

Scallops With Wilted Spinach

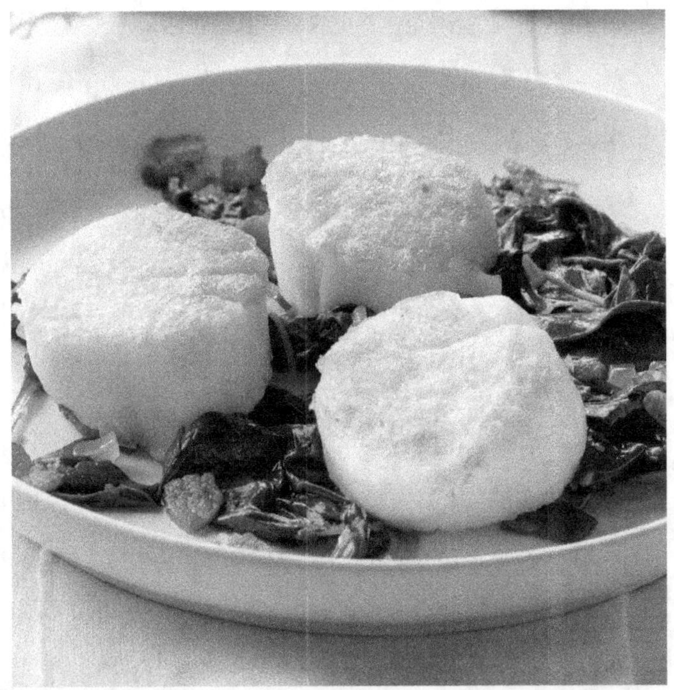

Total Time: 25 min.

Serves: 4

Ingredients

- 4 bacon strips, chopped

- 12 sea scallops (about 1-1/2 pounds), side muscles removed

- 2 shallots, finely chopped

- 1/2 cup white wine or chicken broth

- 8 cups fresh baby spinach (about 8 ounces)

Instructions

1. In a large nonstick skillet, cook bacon over medium heat until crisp, stirring occasionally. Remove with a slotted spoon; drain on paper towels. Discard drippings, reserving 2 tablespoons. Wipe skillet clean if necessary.

2. Pat scallops dry with paper towels. In same skillet, heat 1 tablespoon drippings over medium-high heat. Add scallops; cook until golden brown and firm, 2-3 minutes on each side. Remove from pan; keep warm.

3. Heat remaining drippings in same pan over medium-high heat. Add shallots; cook and stir until tender, 2-3 minutes. Add wine; bring to a boil, stirring to loosen browned bits from pan. Add spinach; cook and stir until wilted, 1-2 minutes. Stir in bacon. Serve with scallops.

Nutrition

- Calories: 247 kcal

- 11g fat

- 12g carbohydrate

- 26g protein.

-

Vegan Falafel

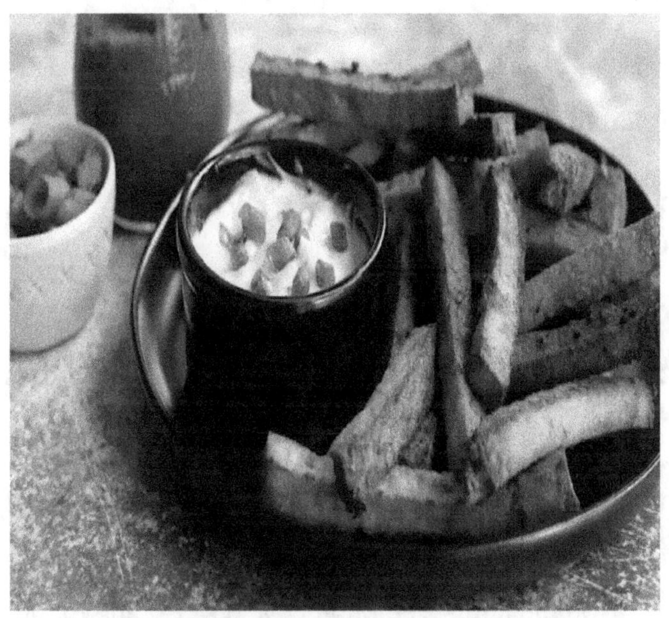

Total Time: 38 minutes

Yield: 12 falafel patties (4 servings)

Ingredients

- 1 cup brined lupini beans

- 1 1/2 cups thawed frozen broccoli

- 1/4 cup tahini

- 2 tbsp lemon juice

- 1 tbsp dried parsley

- 2 tsp cumin

- 2 tbsp ground chia seeds

- 1/2 tsp garlic powder

- 1/4 tsp onion powder

- 1/4 tsp all spice

Instructions

1. Before you start, soak the lupini beans in hot water for between 30-60 minutes and then drain them. This should help to temper some of the overly briney flavor.

2. In a food processor, chop the beans and broccoli until they are in pieces, about the size of a grain of rice (you can even go smaller, if you have the patience!). Transfer this mixture to a medium sized mixing bowl.

3. Add the tahini, lemon juice and seasoning to the mixture and stir until thoroughly combined.

4. Stir in the ground chia seeds completely and let the mixture sit for about 5 minutes, so the chia can absorb some liquid and a thick dough forms.

5. Shape the dough mixture into 12 patties.

6. Arrange the patties in your air fryer in a single layer, and cook at 350F(177C) for 14-15 minutes, depending on how crunchy you like them!

7. Enjoy while warm.

Nutrition

- Calories: 188 kcal

- Fats: 12.2g

- Carbs: 5.1g

- Protein: 11.5g

DINNER RECIPES

Creamy Tuscan Garlic Chicken

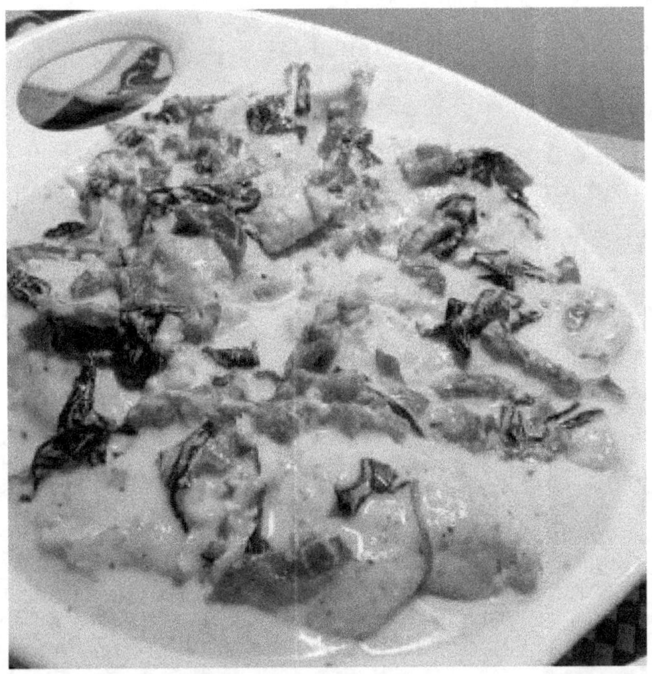

Total Time: 25 Minutes

Servings: 6

Ingredients

- 1½ pounds boneless skinless chicken breasts thinly sliced

- 2 Tablespoons olive oil

- 1 cup heavy cream

- 1/2 cup chicken broth

- 1 teaspoon garlic powder

- 1 teaspoon italian seasoning

- 1/2 cup parmesan cheese

- 1 cup spinach chopped

- 1/2 cup sun dried tomatoes

Instructions

1. In a large skillet add olive oil and cook the chicken on medium high heat for 3-5 minutes on each side or until brown on each side and cooked until no longer pink in center. Remove chicken and set aside on a plate.

2. Add the heavy cream, chicken broth, garlic powder, italian seasoning, and parmesan cheese. Whisk over medium high heat until it starts to thicken. Add the spinach and sundried tomatoes and let it simmer until the spinach starts to wilt. Add the chicken back to the pan and serve over pasta if desired.

Nutrition

- Calories: 368 kcal

- Fat: 25g

- Carbohydrates: 7g

- Protein: 30g

Turkey And Peppers

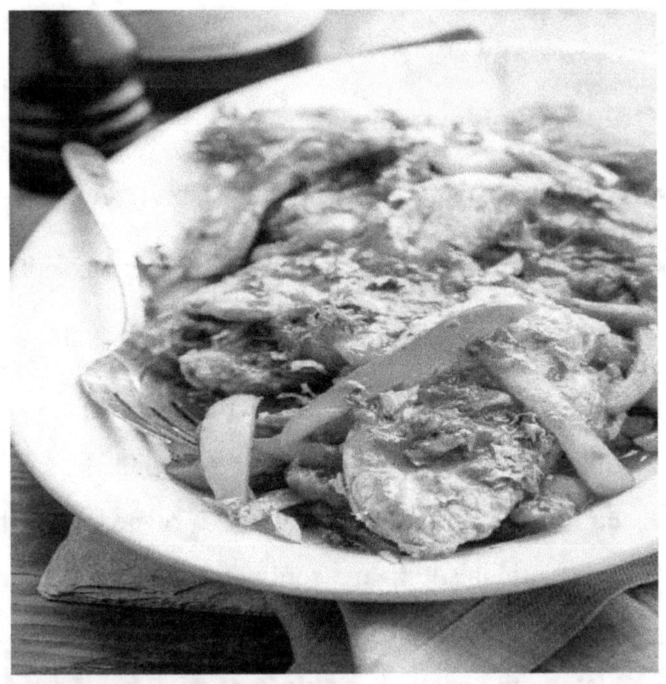

Total Time: 20 Minutes

Serves: 4

Ingredients

- 1 teaspoon salt, divided

- 1 pound turkey tenderloin, cut into thin steaks about ¼-inch thick

- 2 tablespoons extra-virgin olive oil, divided

- ½ large sweet onion, sliced

- 1 red bell pepper, cut into strips

- 1 yellow bell pepper, cut into strips

- ½ teaspoon Italian seasoning

- ¼ teaspoon ground black pepper

- 2 teaspoons red wine vinegar

- 1 14-ounce can crushed tomatoes, preferably fire-roasted

- Chopped fresh parsley and basil for garnish (optional)

Instructions

1. Sprinkle ½ teaspoon salt over turkey. Heat 1 tablespoon oil in a large non-stick skillet over medium high heat. Add half of the turkey and cook, until browned on the bottom, 1 to 3 minutes. Flip and continue cooking until cooked all the way through, 1 to 2 minutes. Remove the turkey to a plate with a slotted spatula, tent with foil to keep warm. Add the remaining 1 tablespoon oil to the skillet, reduce heat to medium and repeat with the remaining turkey, 1 to 3 minutes per side.

2. Add onion, bell peppers and the remaining ½ teaspoon salt to the skillet, cover and cook, removing lid to stir often, until the onion and peppers are softening and brown in spots, 5 to 7 minutes.

3. Remove lid, increase heat to medium high, sprinkle with Italian seasoning and pepper and cook, stirring often until the herbs are fragrant, about 30 seconds. Add vinegar, and

cook, stirring until almost completely evaporated, about 20 seconds. Add tomatoes and bring to a simmer, stirring often.

4. Add the turkey to the skillet with any accumulated juices from the plate and bring to a simmer. Reduce heat to medium-low and cook, turning in the sauce until the turkey is hot all the way through, 1 to 2 minutes. Serve topped with parsley and basil if using.

Nutrition

- Calories: 230 kcal

- Fat: 8g

- Carbohydrates: 11g

- Protein: 30g

Shredded Chicken Chili

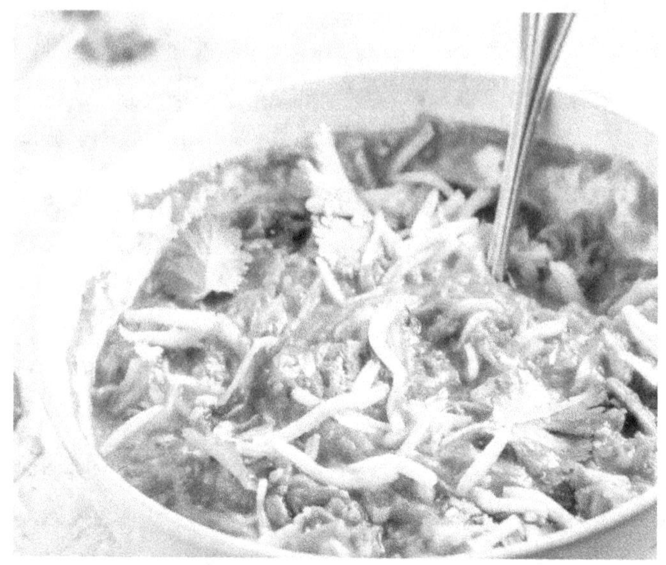

Total Time: 30 minutes

Servings: 6

Ingredients

- 4 chicken breasts large, shredded

- 1 tbsp Butter

- ½ onion chopped

- 2 cups Chicken broth

- 10 oz diced tomatoes canned, undrained

- 2 oz tomato paste

- 1 tbsp Chili powder

- 1 tbsp Cumin

- 1/2 tbsp Garlic powder

- 1 jalapeno pepper chopped (optional)

- 4 oz Cream cheese

- Salt and pepper to taste

Instructions

1. Prepare chicken by boiling chicken breasts in water or broth on stovetop for 10-12 minutes, just barely covered in liquid. Once the meat is no longer pink, remove from fluid and shred with two forks. This same technique can also be used with a pressure cooker at pressure for 5 minutes with a natural release, or a slow cooker for 4-6 hours. Whatever's clever for you! Rotisserie chicken meat can be substituted for the breasts as well.

2. In a large stockpot, melt the butter over medium-high heat. Add the onion and cook until translucent.

3. Add the shredded chicken, chicken broth, diced tomatoes, tomato paste, chili powder, cumin, garlic powder, and jalapeno to the pot and combine by gently stirring over the burner. Bring to a boil, then drop it down to a simmer over medium-low heat and cover for 10 minutes.

4. Cut cream cheese into small, 1-inch chunks.

5. Remove lid and mix in the cream cheese. Increase the

heat back up to medium-high and continue to stir until the cream cheese is completely blended in. Remove from heat and season with salt and pepper to taste.

6. Eat as-is or garnish with toppings of your choice.

Nutrition

- Calories: 201 kcal

- Carbs: 7g

- Protein: 18g

- Fat: 11g

Taco Stuffed Avocados

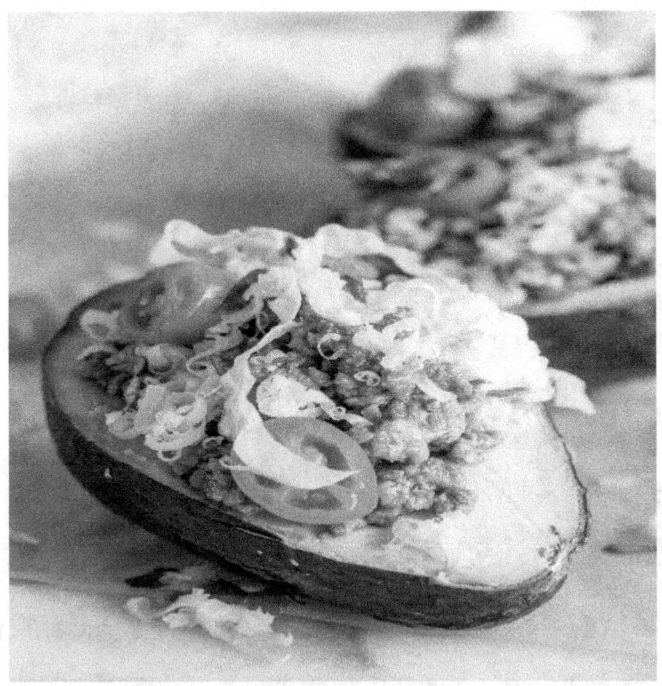

Total Time: 20 Minutes

Serves: 6

Ingredients

- 1 pound ground beef

- 1 tablespoon Chili Powder

- ½ teaspoon Salt

- ¾ teaspoon Cumin

- ½ teaspoon Dried Oregano

- ¼ teaspoon Garlic Powder

- ¼ teaspoon Onion Powder

- 4 ounces tomato sauce

- 3 avocados halved

- 1 cup shredded cheddar cheese

- ¼ cup cherry tomatoes sliced

- ¼ cup lettuce shredded

Additional toppings:

- cilantro

- sour cream

Instructions

1. Add the ground beef to a medium size sauce pan. Cook over medium heat until browned.

2. Drain the grease and add the seasonings and the tomato sauce. Stir to combine. Cook for about 3-4 minutes.

3. Remove the pit from the halved avocados. Load the crater left from the pit with the taco meat. Top with cheese, tomatoes, lettuce, cilantro and sour cream.

4. If you want to make a larger area in the avocado for the toppings, spoon out some of the avocado and set aside to make guacamole! Then fill with toppings.

Nutrition

- Calories: 410 kcal

- Protein: 26g

- Fat: 16g

- Carbs: 5g

Asparagus Stuffed Chicken

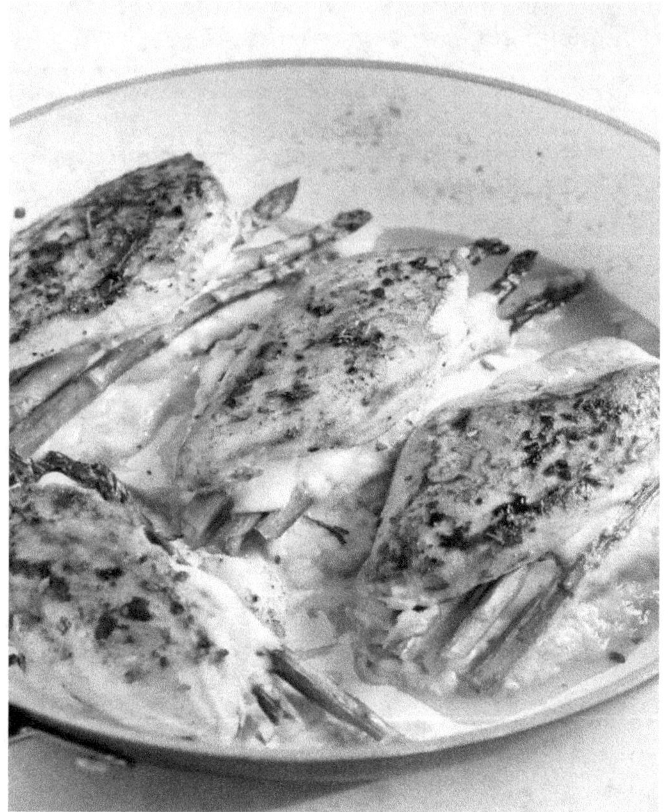

Total Time: 30 minutes

Serves: 3

Ingredients

- 3 Chicken Breasts

- 1 teaspoon Garlic paste

- 12 stalks Asparagus (stalks removed)

- 1/2 cup Cream Cheese

- 1 tablespoon Butter

- 1 teaspoon Olive Oil

- 3/4 cup Marinara Sauce

- 1 cup shredded Mozzarella

- Salt and Pepper to taste

Instructions

1. To start prepping the chicken, butterfly the chicken (or slice it in half without slicing it all the way through. The chicken breast should open out like a butterfly with one end still intact in the middle). Remove the hardy stalks of the asparagus and set aside.

2. Rub salt, pepper and garlic paste all over the chicken breasts (inside and outside). Divide cream cheese between the chicken breasts and spread it on the inside. Place four stalks of asparagus and then fold one side of the breast over the other, tucking it in place with a toothpick to make sure it doesn't come open.

3. Preheat the oven, and set it to broiler. Add butter and olive oil to a hot skillet and place the chicken breasts in it. Cook the breasts on each side for 6-7 minutes (total time will be 14-15 minutes depending on the size of the breast) till the chicken is almost cooked through.

4. Top each breast with 1/4 cup marinara sauce, and divide

the shredded mozzarella on top. Place in the oven and broil for 5 minutes till the cheese melts.

Nutrition

- Calories: 317 kcal

- Total Fat: 20.6g

- Carbs: 11.2g

- Protein: 23.1g

Ground Beef & Cabbage Stir Fry

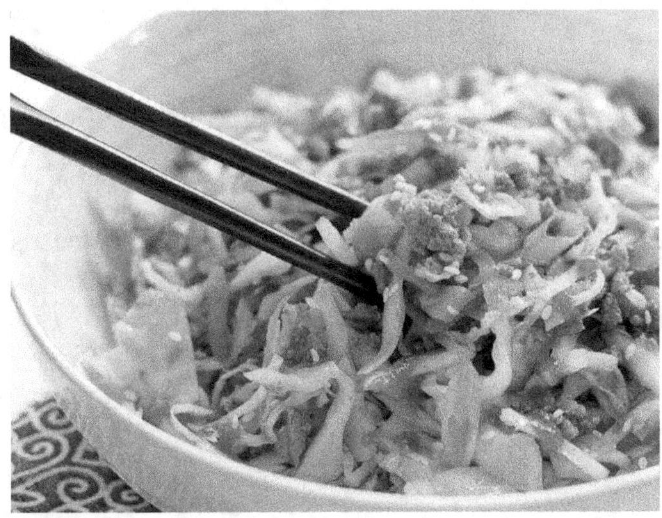

Total Time: 20 mins

Serves: 3

Ingredients

- 1 pound ground beef (I typically use 85% lean)

- 1 (9-ounce) bag coleslaw (or 5 cups mix of shredded fresh cabbage and sliced carrots)

- 2 scallions (also known as green onions), thinly sliced

- 1 tablespoon peeled freshly grated ginger

- 2 tablespoons soy sauce (both regular and low-sodium varieties work well; I use the brand Kikkoman)

- 1 tablespoon sriracha sauce (You can use the brand Huy Fong; can substitute with another chili garlic sauce or your favorite hot sauce)

- (optional) black sesame seeds

Instructions

1. Stir soy sauce and sriracha together with a spoon in a small mixing bowl until smooth; set aside.

2. Prepare a pan large enough to simultaneously hold ground beef and coleslaw; I use a nonstick 10-inch pan with 3-inch-tall sides. No lid needed. It's not necessary to pre-heat the pan, and oil is not required.

3. Add ground beef to the pan over medium-high heat; cook until browned and crumbled, breaking up the meat with a stiff utensil, about 5 minutes. Do not drain fat, which will be used to fry coleslaw in the next step.

4. Keeping beef in the pan, stir in coleslaw mix. Cook until cabbage is wilted and tender, stirring frequently, about 5 minutes.

5. Reduce heat to medium-low. Stir in prepared sauce (soy sauce and sriracha) and ginger until well-mixed, about 1 minute.

6. Turn off the heat. Stir in sliced scallions, and optionally garnish with sesame seeds. Serve while hot.

7. Leftovers: Cover and store leftovers in the refrigerator for up to a few days. Reheat using the microwave or on the

stovetop until warmed through.

Nutrition

- Calories: 420 kcal

- Total Fat: 22g

- Net Carb: 6g

- Protein: 39g

Loaded Cauliflower

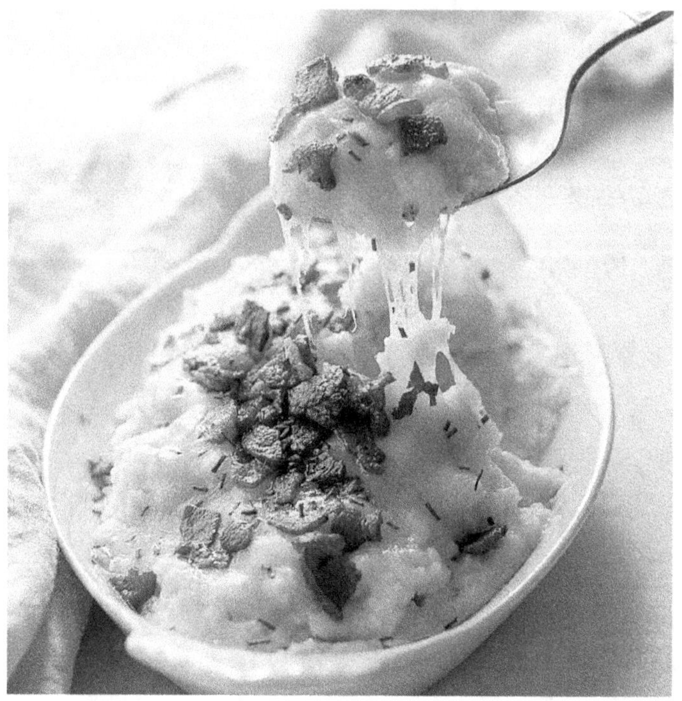

Total Time: 20 minutes

Servings: 4

Ingredients

- 1 pound cauliflower

- 4 ounces sour cream

- 1 cup grated cheddar cheese

- 2 slices bacon cooked and crumbled

- 2 tablespoons chives snipped

- 3 tablespoons butter

- 1/4 teaspoon garlic powder

- salt and pepper to taste

Instructions

1. Cut the cauliflower into florettes and add them to a microwave safe bowl. Add 2 tablespoons of water and cover with cling film. Microwave for 5-8 minutes, depending on your microwave, until completely cooked and tender. Drain the excess water and let sit uncovered for a minute or two. (Alternately, steam your cauliflower the conventional way. You may need to squeeze a little water out of the cauliflower after cooking.)

2. Add the cauliflower to a food processor and process until fluffy. Add the butter, garlic powder, and sour cream and process until it resembles the consistency of mashes potatoes. Remove the mashed cauliflower to a bowl and add most of the chives, saving some to add to the top later. Add half of the cheddar cheese and mix by hand. Season with salt and pepper.

3. Top the loaded cauliflower with the remaining cheese, remaining chives and bacon. Put back into the microwave to melt the cheese or place the cauliflower under the broiler for a few minutes.

Nutrition

- Calories: 298 kcal

- Carbohydrates: 7.4g

- Protein: 11.6g

- Fat: 24.6g

Salmon Patties With Lime Juice

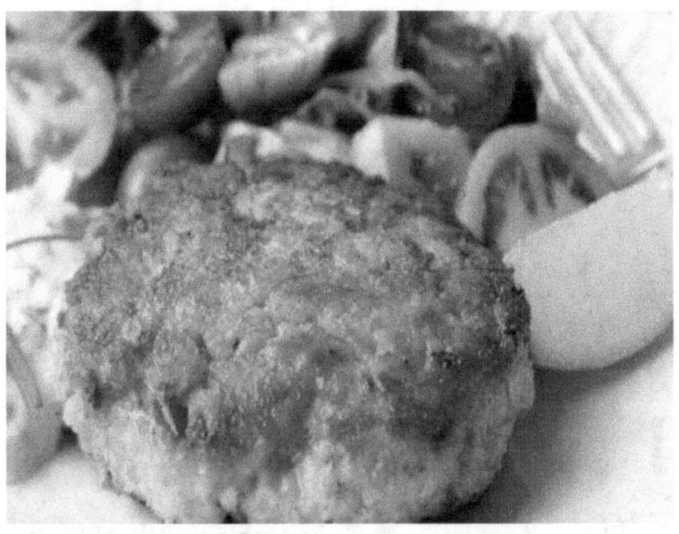

Total: 20 minutes

Servings: 6 patties

Ingredients

- 6 tablespoons water

- 2 tablespoons golden flaxseed meal

- 18 oz Wild Pink Salmon (about 3 cans), well drained (see notes)

- ½ cup almond meal

- 1/2 cup fresh parsley ,chopped

- 1 shallot ,finely chopped

- 1 green onion ,sliced

- 1 teaspoon salt

- 1 teaspoon garlic powder

- ½ teaspoon dill

- ¼ teaspoon black pepper

- 2 tablespoons lime juice

- 2 tablespoons olive oil

Instructions

1. Add flaxseed meal and water to a small bowl and stir. Let rest for 5 minutes to thicken.

2. Flake the salmon apart in a medium bowl. Add almond meal, parsley, shallot, green onion, salt, garlic powder, dill, black pepper, lime juice, and the flaxseed mixture. Mix until well incorporated.

3. Form into 6 patties. I use a ½ cup measuring cup to portion the mixture and to make sure all the patties are the same size.

4. Heat olive oil over medium heat in a nonstick skillet. Fry the patties for 4- 5 minutes on each side until golden brown and crispy.

5. Serve with cilantro lime cauliflower rice, if desired

Nutrition

- Calories: 232 kcal

- Carbohydrates: 4g

- Protein: 22g

- Fat: 14g

Salmon Gremolata Recipe & Roasted Vegetables

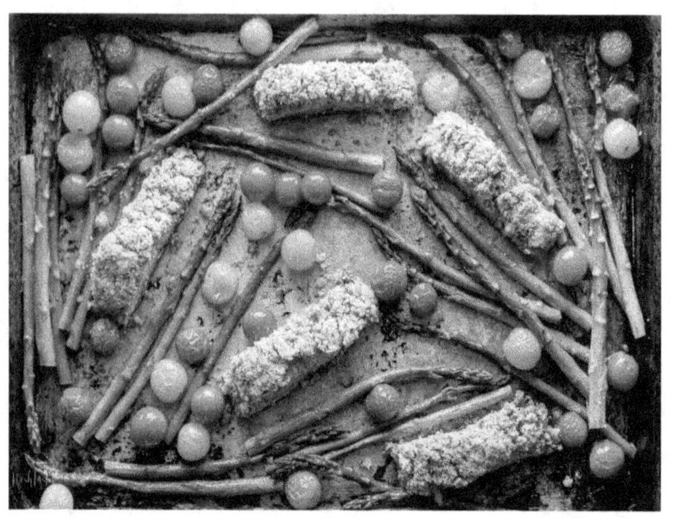

Total Time: 30 minutes

Total Carbs: 12 g

Serves: 4

Ingredients

- 4 salmon fillets

Gremolata

- 2 cloves garlic

- 1/4 cup parsley leaves

- 1 lemon, zested

- 1 cup almond flour

- 1 tbsp olive oil

- salt

- pepper

Roasted Vegetables (Optional)

- 1 bunch asparagus

- 1 cup cherry tomatoes

- 1 tbsp olive oil

- salt

- pepper

Instructions

1. Heat your oven to 350F for a fan oven, 380F for non fan oven.

2. Blitz the garlic, parsley and almond meal together in a blender or food processor, then stir in the lemon zest.

3. Place the salmon fillets on a greased or parchment lined sheet pan.

4. Season the salmon fillets with salt and pepper, brush or spray with a little oil, then carefully press the Gremolata crumb mixture on top.

5. If you are using the optional vegetables to roast alongside the salmon, simply toss them in a little oil, place them around the salmon on the sheet pan and season with salt

and pepper.

6. Bake for 15-20 mins until the fish is cooked through and the tops are golden.

Nutrition

- Calories: 494 kcal

- Fat: 31g

- Carbs: 12g

- Protein: 42g

Portobello Mushroom "Tacos"

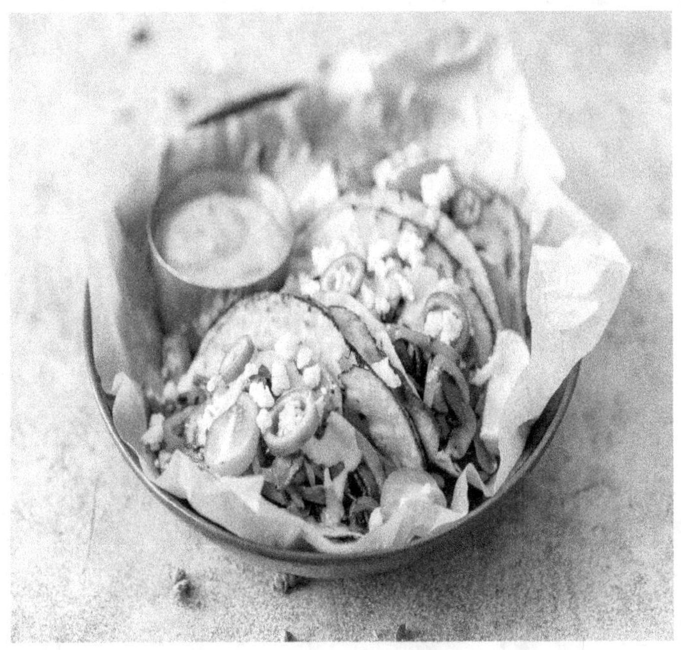

Serves: 6

Total Time: 20 min

Ingredients

Portobello Mushrooms

- 1 pound (450g) portobello mushrooms

- 1/4 cup (60g) spicy harissa, or use a mild harissa

- 3 tablespoons olive oil, divided

- 1 teaspoon ground cumin

- 1 teaspoon onion powder

- 6 collard green leaves

Guacamole

- 2 medium ripe avocados

- 2 tablespoons chopped tomatoes

- 2 tablespoons chopped red onion

- 1 1/2 to 2 tablespoons lemon or lime juice

- pinch of salt

- 1 tablespoon chopped cilantro

Optional Toppings

- cashew cream

- chopped tomatoes

- chopped cilantro

Instructions

1. Remove the stem of the portobellos. Rinse mushrooms and pat dry.

2. Mix harissa, 1 1/2 tablespoons olive oil, cumin, and onion powder in a bowl. Brush each mushroom with the harissa mixture, making sure to cover the edges of the mushroom as well. Let mushroom marinade for 15 minutes.

3. While the mushrooms are marinating, prepare guacamole. Halve and pit the avocados and scoop out the

flesh. Mash avocados and mix in chopped tomatoes, red onion, lemon (or lime) juice, salt, and cilantro. Set aside.

4. Rinse collard greens. Chop off the tough stems and set aside.

5. When the mushrooms are done marinating, heat 1 1/2 tablespoons of olive oil in a skillet or sauté pan over medium-high heat. Place the portobello mushrooms in the pan and cook for 3 minutes. Flip over and cook for another 2 to 3 minutes. Each side should be browned.

6. Turn off the heat and let the mushrooms rest for 2 to 3 minutes before slicing.

7. Take a collard green leaf and fill it with a few slices of portobello. Add guacamole, chopped tomatoes, cashew cream, and cilantro to your liking.

Nutrition

- Calories: 405 kcal

- Total Fat 34.4g

- Total Carbohydrate: 24g

- Protein 10g

30-Minute Sesame Ginger Meatball Soup

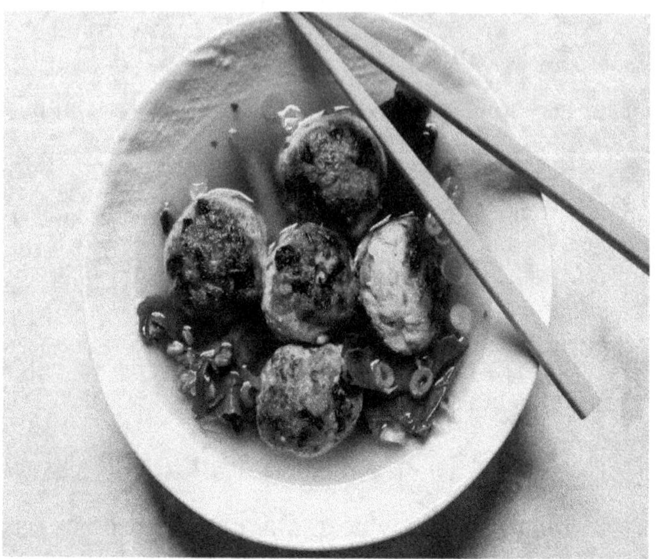

Total Time: 30 minutes

Servings: 3

Equipment: Air-fryer

Ingredients

- 1 teaspoon grated ginger

- 2 garlic cloves, finely minced

- 2 teaspoons yellow or white onion, finely minced

- 2 tablespoons chopped organic cilantro (plus more for garnish)

- 3 teaspoons coconut aminos

- 1 pound 85/15 grass-fed ground beef

- 15 ounces baby boy choy, quartered lengthwise

- ½ pound shiitake mushrooms, sliced

- ½ teaspoon kosher salt

- ¾ cup Primal Kitchen Sesame Ginger Dressing

- Sesame seeds to garnish

Instructions

1. Mix ginger, garlic, onion, cilantro, coconut aminos and beef together in a large bowl.

2. Shape into nine meatballs.

3. Tear three large sheets of foil or parchment paper (about 6 inches wide each).

4. Divide bok choy and mushrooms evenly in the center of the 3 slices of foil or paper.

5. Place 3 meatballs in each pack.

6. Curl up the sides of the foil or paper a bit, and place packs into the AirFryer basket, on a sheet tray or in a casserole dish.

7. Pour ¼ cup of Sesame Ginger Dressing inside each pack.

8. Roll the edges of each pack to seal the packets and ensure

there are no holes openings in the packs.

9. Use the AirFryer's convection oven Bake setting, slide the basket with the packets into the oven. Bake for 20 minutes.

10. Remove from AirFryer and carefully open packets.

11. Pour contents of packets into bowls.

12. Garnish each bowl with a few fresh cilantro sprigs and a sprinkle of sesame seeds.

Nutritional

- Calories: 489 kcal

- Net Carbs: 7.6 grams

- Fat: 29.4 grams

- Protein: 44 grams

Meatballs With Himalayan Salt & Black Pepper

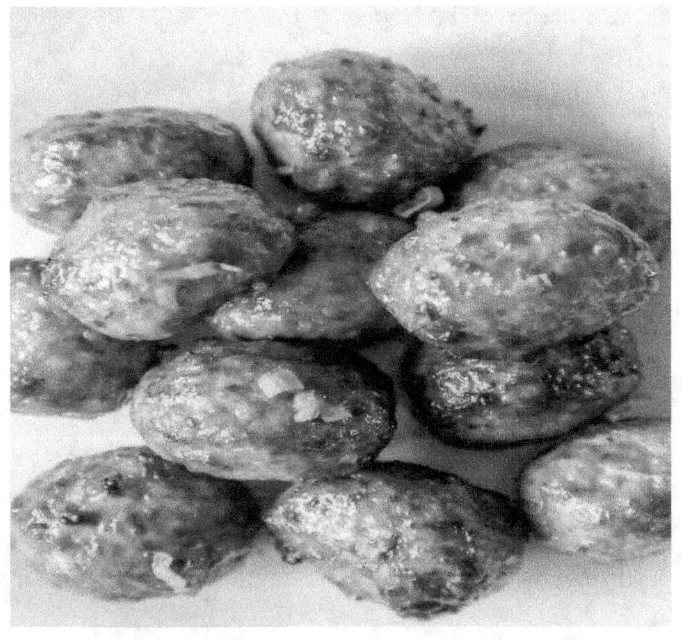

Total Time: 22 min

Serves: 4

Equipment: Air-fryer

Ingredients

- 1 lb ground beef 85/15

- 1/3 cup crushed pork rinds

- 1/4 cup scallions, chopped

- 2 cloves garlic, minced

- 2 tbsp coconut aminos/soy sauce

- 1 tbsp cilantro, finely chopped

- 2 tsp fish sauce (optional)

- 1/2 tsp Sriracha Sauce

- 1 tsp ground ginger

- 1 tsp pink himalayan salt

- 1/2 tsp black pepper

Instructions

1. Preheat your air fryer at 350 for 2-3 minutes.

2. Combine all ingredients in a large bowl and mix thoroughly using your hands.

3. Form the meat into 16 1.5-inch balls and set on a plate.

4. Add meatballs to air fryer basket, making sure they don't touch or over crowd the basket (work in batches if needed.)

5. Cook in air fryer for 10-12 minutes at 350 degrees.

6. Remove from the air fryer and serve immediately.

Nutrition

- Net Carbs: 2g

- Calories 313

- Fat 23g

- Protein 22

Crispy & Pepperish Pork Belly Crack

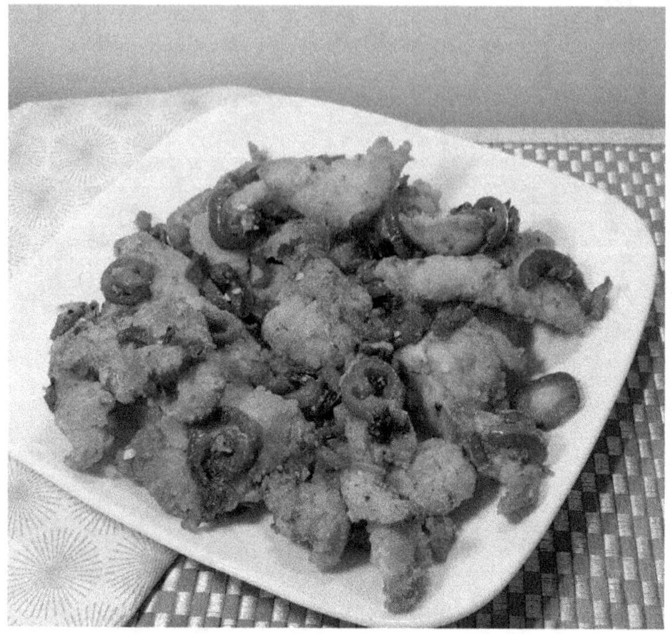

These pork belly slices cook up perfectly in the air fryer.

Total Time: 20 Minutes

Serves: 4

Equipment: Air-fryer

Ingredients

- 1 lb raw sliced pork belly strips

- 1 teaspoon sea salt

- 1/2 teaspoon pepper

Instructions

1. Cut pork belly slices into bite sized pieces with scissors

2. Toss pieces in a bowl with salt and pepper

3. Preheat air fryer for 3 minutes

4. Place pieces into air fryer at 390 for 15 minutes, checking and turning at 5 minute intervals so they get crispy all over

5. Depending on thickness of slices, they should be fully cooked in 15 minutes

6. Drain on paper towels

7. Enjoy!

Nutrition

- Calories: 332 kcal

- Total Fat: 24g

- Carbohydrates: 0g

- Protein: 26g

Turkey Meatballs With Fresh Cilantro

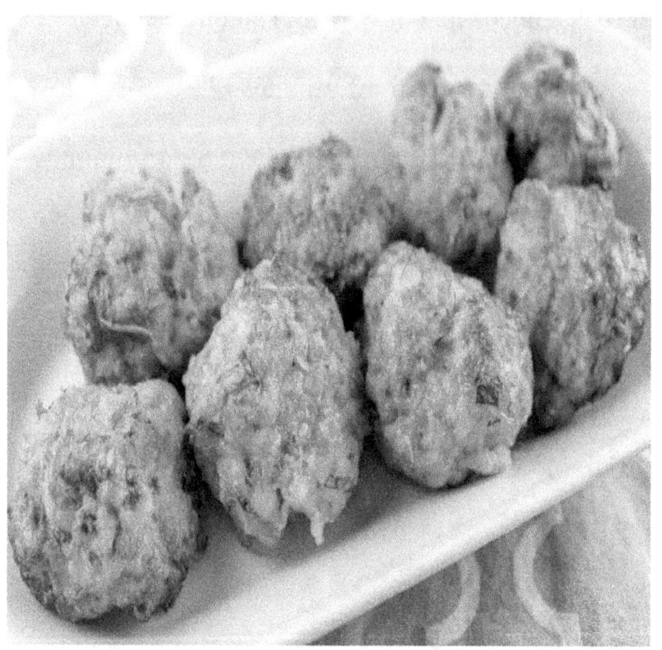

These easy Air Fryer Turkey Meatballs are sure to be a family favourite.

Total Time: 15 mins

Servings: 4

Equipment: Air-fryer

Ingredients

- 1.5 lb turkey mince

- 1 red bell pepper, deseeded and finely chopped

- 1 large egg lightly beaten

- 4 tablespoons minced fresh herbs parsley

- 1 tablespoon minced fresh cilantro coriander

- Salt

- Black pepper

Instructions

1. Preheat air fryer to 400F / 200C.

2. Mix all the ingredients (minus the cooking spray) together in a bowl.

3. Shape into 1-1/4-in meatballs.

4. Place half the meatballs a single layer in air fryer basket; cook for 7-10 mins until lightly browned and cooked through (shaking halfway through).

5. Remove and keep warm, and repeat with the remaining meatballs.

6. Serve warm with toothpicks and a dipping sauce.

Turkey Meatballs Tips

1. Try and make sure the meatballs are all a similar size so that they cook at the same time.

2. Make the meatballs smallish so that they hold together during cooking.

Nutrition

- Calories: 220 kcal

- Carbohydrates: 2g

- Protein: 42g

- Fat: 4g

Avocado Fries Made With Lemon Juice - Oven & Air-fryer Versions

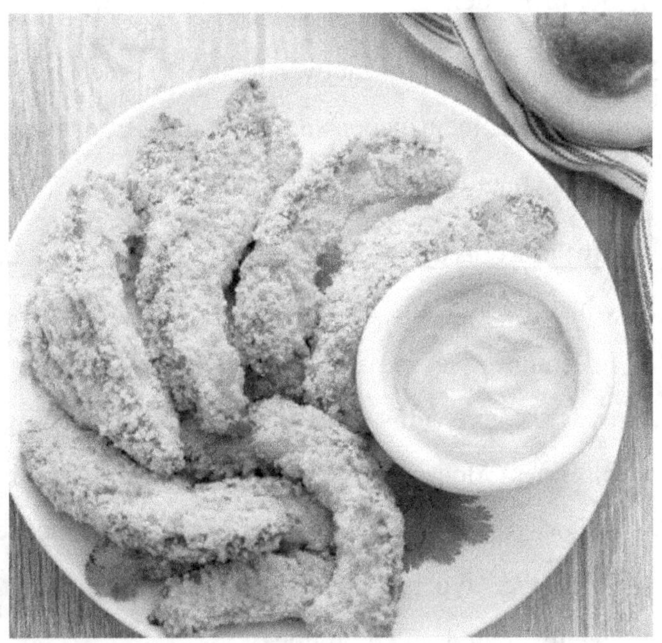

Total Time: 25 min

Serves: 5

Ingredients

- 2 large firm and ripe avocados peeled and pitted

- juice of one lemon

- 1 large egg whisked

- 1 cup superfine blanched almond flour

- 1 cup grated parmesan cheese

- cooking oil spray

Instructions

1. Slice avocado into thick wedges/slices, about 1/2 inch to 3/4 inch thick.

2. If baking fries, preheat oven to 400°F. Line a baking sheet with parchment paper and set aside. If not baking, skip this step and move on to the next step.

3. **<u>Optional Step:</u>** To cut some of the bitterness that occurs when the avocado is cooked, you can coat the avocados in lemon juice and also squeeze more fresh lemon juice over the avocados after they are done cooking. If the bitterness doesn't bother you, you can skip this step. Otherwise, add avocado slices to a bowl. Squeeze lemon juice over avocados. Gently toss avocado until they are evenly coated in lemon juice.

4. Assemble your coating ingredients. In a small bowl add whisked egg. Add almond flour and cheese to food processor and pulse until evenly mixed and parmesan cheese resembles coarse grains of sand. Pour into a medium bowl.

5. Line the part of your work station where you will be coating the avocado with parchment paper. Spoon a small amount of breading onto the parchment paper (just enough to cover the bottom of an avocado slice).

6. Dip an avocado slice in the egg wash. After it is fully coated, shake it a few times, making sure to shake off any excess egg drippings back into the egg bowl before adding it to the breading. The reason for doing this is that you don't want the egg drippings going into the breading. The moisture will cause the breading to clump and they will no longer stick.

7. Place the avocado slice onto the small mound of breading, applying a little pressure so those breading sticks to the bottom of the avocado.

8. Wipe your hand that was holding the avocado so that your hand is also dry before touching the breading. Sprinkle breading over the surface of the avocado, until it is coated in crumbs. Use your fingers to gently press the breading onto the avocado so that it sticks. This works better than rolling the avocado in breading.

9. Carefully set the avocado slice onto your prepared baking sheet if baking or into the air fryer basket if you are using the air fryer. Repeat with remaining avocado slices. Make sure to place avocado fries in a single layer in basket or on baking sheet so they do not overlap or touch.

10. Spray surface of avocado fries with cooking oil spray.

11. Oven: bake in preheated oven until coating is crispy, about 25 minutes.

12. Air Fryer: set temperature of air fryer to 375°F and cook for about 10 minutes or until coating is dark golden brown and crispy.

13. If desired, squeeze fresh lemon juice onto fries. Serve immediately while still crispy. You can serve mine with spicy mayonnaise which you can make by mixing mayonnaise with hot sauce. You can also garnished with some fresh cilantro.

Nutrition

- Calories: 371kcal

- Carbohydrates: 4g

- Protein: 15g

- Fat: 30g

Crispy Garlic Croutons

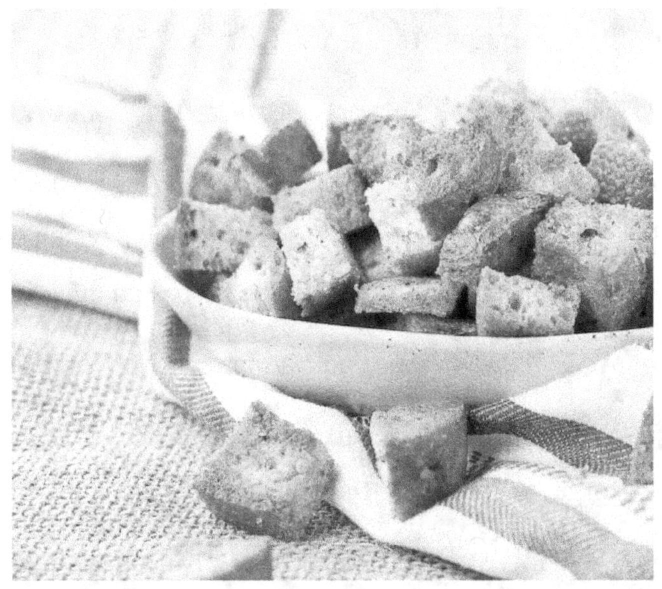

Crispy Garlic Keto Croutons Recipe made in an Air Fryer are not only delicious to make, but also done in just a few minutes.

Equipment: Air-fryer

Total Time: 20 Minutes

Serves: 10

Ingredients

- 2 Cups of Keto Farmers Bread half of the loaf

- 1 Tbsp of Marjoram

- 2Tbsp Olive Oil

- 1/2 Tbsp Garlic Powder

Instructions

1. **Keto Farmers Bread is used in this recipe.**

2. Make sure your bread is cooled. Cut it into same size slices and then squares.

3. Place all of the croutons into a big bowl, which would be spacious enough to mix all the herbs and oil.

4. Add oil, Dry Garlic and Marjoram.

5. With a big spatula, mix all of the croutons fully. Do not forget to make sure the oil and herbs are spread evenly.

6. Depending on your Air Fryer, fill it up with your Keto Croutons. Make sure you only add one layer, otherwise they will not crisp fully.

7. Switch the Air Fryer on, temperature of 400 degress. You do not need to add additional oil, since you have already coated your Keto Croutons with oil before. In just 10 minutes, the croutons will be done fully.

8. After 10 minutes the Crunchy Keto Croutons are ready to be served. Let them cool or serve them still hot or warm.

9. Enjoy!

Nutrition

- Calories: 50 kcal

- Total Fat: 4g

- Carbohydrates: 1g

- Protein: 2g

DESSERTS

Keto Butter Pecan Cheesecake

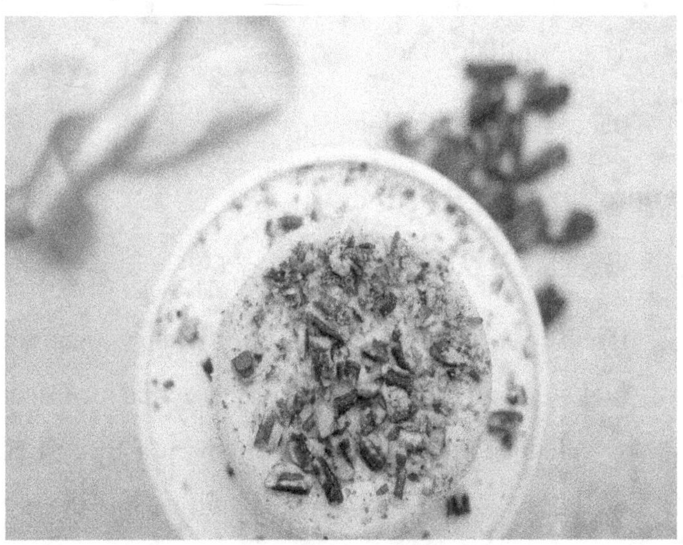

Serves:

Ingredients

Cheesecake crust

- 1 tbsp salted butter, melted

- 4 tbsp pecans, finely crushed

- ½ tbsp powdered erythritol

Filling

- 4 tbsp butter

- 8 oz. cream cheese, softened

- 4 tbsp powdered erythritol

- 2 tbsp unsweetened almond milk or heavy whipping

cream

- 1 egg, beaten

- 1 tsp vanilla extract

- pecans, for garnishing

Instructions

1. Preheat the oven to 350°F (175°C).

2. Grease a 4-inch (10 cm) springform pan with butter. Place melted butter, crushed pecans and confectioner's sweetener in a small bowl. Stir with a fork to combine well. Use your fingers to press mixture into the bottom of the springform pan.

3. Place in oven to pre-bake for 6 minutes while you prepare the filling.

4. Place the butter in a small saucepan over medium-high heat. Stirring often, heat until the butter foams up and brown (but not black!) flecks appear. Remove from the heat and allow to cool a bit. This brown butter creates a caramel-like flavor to the cheesecake.

5. Place softened cream cheese, confectioner's sweetener, almond milk or cream, egg and vanilla in a medium bowl. Use a hand mixer to combine well.

6. Slowly add the browned butter and stir to combine. Pour mixture into pre-baked shell. Tent loosely with foil and

bake for 30-35 minutes or until cheesecake is set and barely jiggles in the center.

7. Remove from oven and allow to chill for 10 minutes then place in fridge to chill for at least 2 hours.

Nutrition

- Net carbs: 4 g kcal

- Fat: 39 g

- Protein: 6 g

- Calories: 383 kcal

Keto Waffles With Blueberry Butter

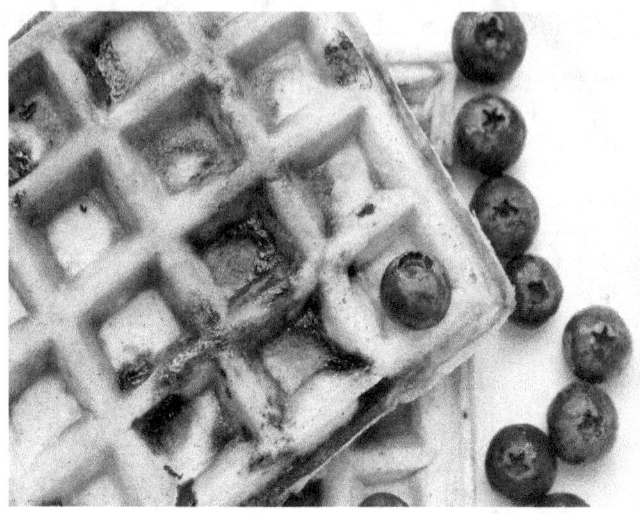

Total Time: 20 min

Serves: 4

Ingredients

- 5 oz. melted butter

- 8 eggs

- 1 tsp vanilla extract

- 2 tsp baking powder

- 1/3 cup coconut flour

- Blueberry Butter

- 3 oz. butter

- 1 oz. fresh blueberries

Instructions

1. Mix melted butter and eggs. Add remaining ingredients and mix to a smooth batter using an electric hand mixer.

2. Allow to rest for 5 minutes while you heat the waffle iron to medium.

3. After properly heated, pour batter into iron and bake until golden. Baking time depends on the size of your waffle iron; I filled mine with 3/4 cup batter. Repeat with remaining batter.

4. Mix butter and blueberries with an electric hand mixer and serve with waffles.

Nutrition

- Calories: 575 kcal

- Net carbs: 3 g

- Fat: 56 g

- Protein: 14 g

Cannoli Sheet Cake

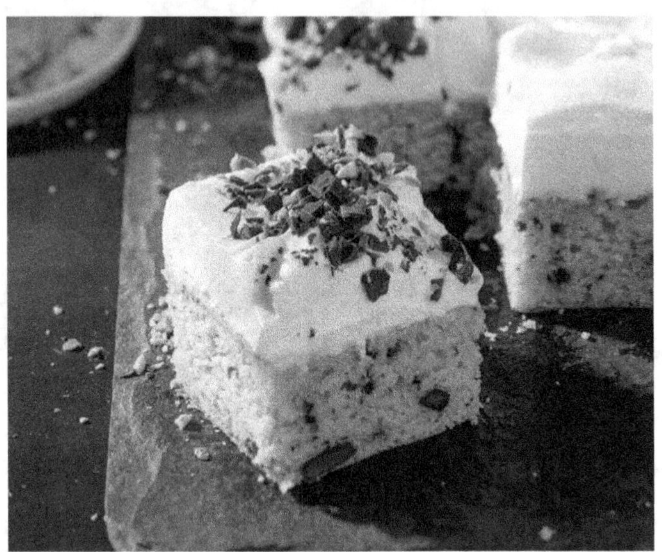

Total Time: 47 mins

Serves: 20

Ingredients

Sheet Cake:

- 2 cups almond flour

- 2/3 cup Swerve Sweetener

- 1/3 cup coconut flour

- 1/3 cup whey protein powder (can also use egg white protein powder)

- 1 tbsp baking powder

- 1/2 tsp salt

* 3 large eggs

* 1/2 cup butter (melted and cooled)

* 2/3 cup water

* 1 tsp vanilla extract

Cannoli Cream Frosting:

* 3/4 cup whole milk ricotta (room temperature)

* 4 ounces cream cheese (softened)

* 1/2 cup powdered Swerve Sweetener

* 1 1/4 cups heavy whipping cream (divided)

* 1/2 tsp vanilla extract

* 1/3 cup sugar-free mini chocolate chips (or regular sugar-free chocolate chips)

* Additional powdered sweetener for sprinkling

Instructions

Cake:

1. Preheat the oven to 325F and grease a 10x15 jelly roll pan very well. You can also do this in an 11x17 pan but it will be thinner and will bake faster.

2. In a large bowl, whisk together the almond flour, sweetener, coconut flour, whey protein, baking powder, and salt. Stir in the eggs, melted butter, water, and vanilla extract until well combined.

3. Spread the batter as evenly as possible in the prepared pan and bake 18 to 22 minutes, until golden brown and just firm to the touch. Remove and let cool completely.

4. Cannoli Frosting:

5. In a food processor or high powered blender, combine the ricotta and the cream cheese. Blend briefly until well combined. Add the sweetener, 1/4 cup of the heavy cream, and the vanilla extract. Blend until smooth.

6. In a large bowl, beat the remaining 1 cup of cream until it holds stiff peaks. Add the ricotta mixture and fold together until well combined. Spread over the cooled cake.

7. Sprinkle with the chocolate chips and refrigerate at least 1 hour to set. Sprinkle with additional powdered sweetener just before serving.

Nutrition

- Calories: 235 kcal

- Fat: 20g

- Carbs: 6.2g

- Protein: 6.8g

Funfetti Cookies

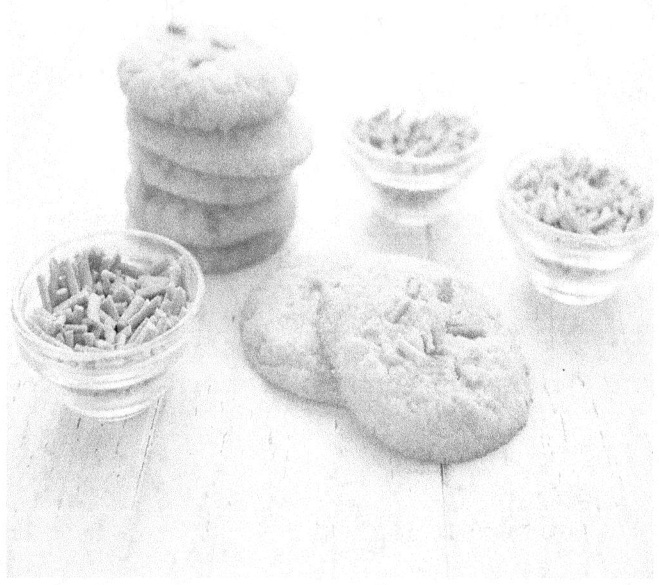

Total Time: 38 mins

Serves: 12

Ingredients

Cookies:

- 1/2 cup butter softened

- 2/3 cup Swerve Sweetener

- 1 large egg room temperature

- 1/2 tsp vanilla extract

- 1/2 tsp cake batter flavoring (optional, see recipe notes)

- 2 cups almond flour

- 1 1/2 tsp baking powder

- 1/4 tsp salt

- 1/3 cup sugar-free sprinkles divided

Frosting:

- 4 ounces cream cheese softened

- 3 tbsp butter softened

- 1/4 cup powdered Swerve Sweetener

- 2 to 3 tbsp heavy whipping cream room temperature

- 1/2 tsp vanilla extract

- 2 tbsp sugar-free sprinkles

-

Instructions

Cookies:

1. Preheat the oven to 325F and line 2 cookie sheets with silicone mats or parchment paper.

2. In a large bowl, beat the butter with the sweetener until well combined and fluffy. Add the egg, vanilla, and cake batter flavor, if using, and beat until well combined.

3. Add the almond flour, baking powder, and salt and beat until the dough comes together. Gently stir in the sugar-free sprinkles.

4. Roll the dough into 1 inch balls and space about 2 inches apart on the prepared baking sheets. Press each ball down to about 1/2 inch thick with the heel of your hand.

5. Bake 15 to 18 minutes, until just golden around the edges, switching the pans halfway through baking. They will still be a bit soft. Remove and let cool on the pans.

Frosting:

1. Beat the cream cheese and butter together until smooth. Beat in the powdered sweetener, then beat in the cream and vanilla extract.

2. Spread over the cooled cookies and sprinkle with additional sprinkles.

Nutrition

- Calories: 262 kcal
- Fat: 24g
- Carbs: 5.1g
- Protein 5.5g

No Bake Cookies

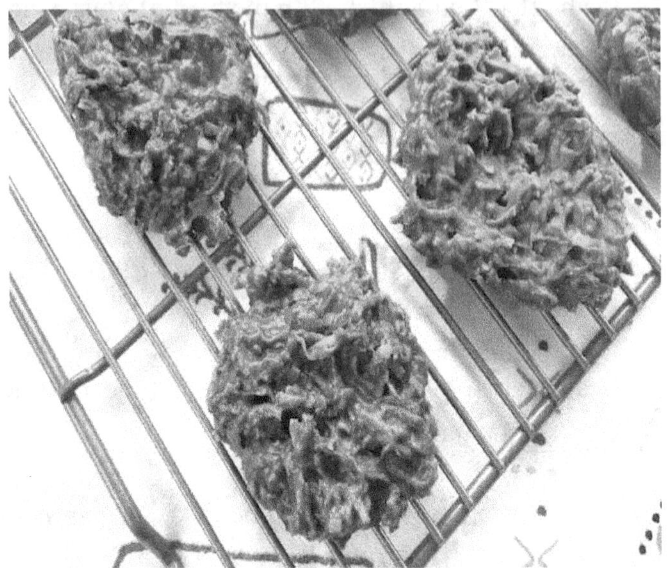

Total Time: 30 mins

Servings: 20

Ingredients

- 1 1/3 cups creamy peanut butter

- 2 teaspoons vanilla extract

- 2 Tablespoons cocoa powder unsweetened

- 2 cups coconut flakes unsweetened

- 2 Tablespoons butter melted

- 1 teaspoon erythritol (optional)

Instructions

1. Prepare a large baking sheet with parchment paper or a non-stick silicone baking mat.

2. In a large mixing bowl, combine the peanut butter, vanilla extract, melted butted, coconut flake and cocoa powder and stir until well combined. (If you like your cookies a little sweeter, feel free to add 1-2 teaspoons of your favorite sugar-alternative. I used Swerve.)

3. Scoop batter onto your prepared baking sheet. Use the back of the spoon to gently shape each scoop into into a 3" cookie.

4. Place in freezer for 30 minutes to set.

5. Store in an airtight container in the freezer.

Nutrition

- Calories: 153kcal

- Fat: 13g

- Carbohydrates: 5g

- Fiber: 1g

- Protein: 4g

OUTLOOK

Intermittent Fasting offers a host of unique benefits that cannot be ignored if you want to stay healthy for a long period of time.

You need to make sure you are eating enough and taking in the right nutrients!

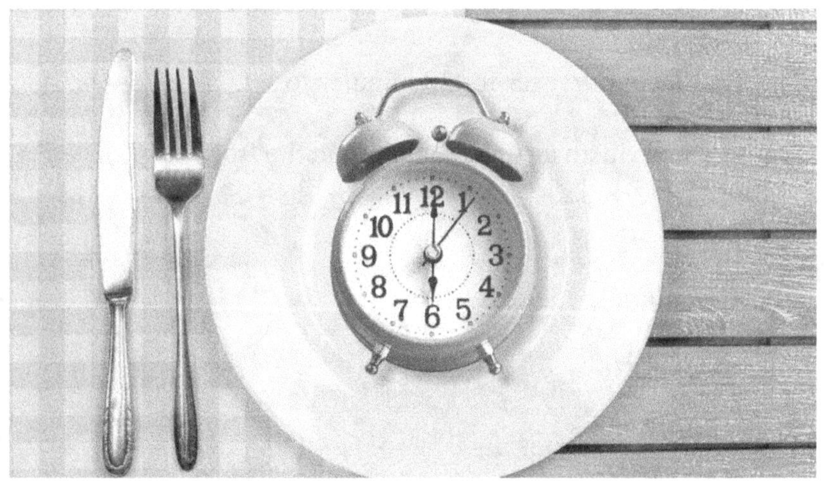

Did you enjoy this cookbook? Kindly let me know by rating your experience and sharing your thoughts with me!

Stay Healthy!!!

Ella

xo-xo

www.ingramcontent.com/pod-product-compliance
Lightning Source LLC
Chambersburg PA
CBHW070706250726
48662CB00001B/276